Neuroscience
The Most Rapid Review of All Topics

Dr. Timur M. Urakov

Timur M. Urakov

Copyright © 2018 Timur M. Urakov

All rights reserved.

ISBN-13: 978-1987440638
ISBN-10: 1987440633
:

NEUROSCIENCE: The Most Rapid Review Of All Topics

HOW TO USE THIS BOOK

This book contains all key terms of neuroscience outlined in a concise systematic manner. The chapters are around a page long to allow for quick glance of an entire topic. Before this book is used it is implied that the reader has studied the subject in a more comprehensive text. If any of the terms do not trigger a memory the reader should go back to their expanded sources for further review.

CONTENTS

Module A. Neuroanatomy

1. Basic CNS organization
2. Basic Neuroimaging
3. General Morphology
4. Brain Surface
5. Meninges and Arteries
6. Ventricles, CSF, Veins, Sinuses
7. Brainstem/Cerebellum

Module B. Cellular Neuroscience

8. Neurons/Glia
9. Resting Excitable cells.
10. Stimulated Excitable Cells
11. AP Initiation & Conduction
12. Synaptic Transmission in Spinal Cord
13. Neuromuscular Transmission
14. Transmitter release
15. Neurotransmitter systems
16. Transport within CNS

Module C. Development

17. Nervous System Development

Module D. Sensory Systems

18. Sensory systems. Overview
19. Somatosensory System
20. Touch
21. PAIN
22. Visual System
23. The Retina
24. Visual Pathways
25. Eye Movement
26. Vestibular System
27. Ocular Reflexes
28. Auditory System
29. Chemical Senses

Module E. Motor Systems

30. Organization of the Motor System
31. Corticospinal & Corticobulbar fibers
32. Other Motor Pathways

33. Muscle Innervation & Motor Unit.
34. Diseases of the NMJ & Motor Unit.
35. PNS disorders
36. Spinal Reflexes

Module F. Movement Disorders

37. Movement Disorders: Intro
38. Movement Disorders: Basal Ganglia
39. Movement Disorders: Cerebellum

Module G. ANS

40. Autonomic Nervous System
41. Hypothalamus
42. Autonomic Control Circuits

Module H. Selected topics

43. Sexual Differentiation of the Brain
44. Emotions
45. Consciousness
46. Language and Aphasias
47. Mental Illness
48. Addiction
49. EEG & Epilepsy
50. Sleep
51. Memory Systems

BONUS: Relevant topics in Anatomy

53. ANS General Overview
54. ANS of Head Neck
55. Overview of Cranial Nerves
56. Cranial Nerves V and VII
57. Face & Scalp
58. Nasal cavity, Pterygopalatine fossa
59. Infratemporal Fossa
60. Orbit and Eye
61. Triangles of the neck
62. Autonomics of Abdomen
63. Pelvic Vessels & Nerves
64. Development: Blastocyst & Bilaminar disk. Gastrulation/Somites
65. Development of Brain
66. Development of Ear
67. Development of Eye

NEUROSCIENCE: The Most Rapid Review Of All Topics

Module A. Neuroanatomy.

1. Basic CNS organization.

1. Above **midbrain** – ventral-dorsal turn 90 degrees – developmental brain fold
2. ANS: Sns, Pns, **Enteric NS**
3. Boundary between CNS and PNS: **Redlich-Obersteiner's zone** – myelin sheaths are thin./ last node of Ranvier before spinal cord at entry of Dorsal root.
4. 5 parts: **Telencephalon** (Cortex+most of Basal ganglia; lateral ventricles), **Diencephalon** (Thalamus+Hypothalamus+Pituitary+Mammillary bodies; 3rd ventricle), **Mesencephalon** (Midbrain+Cerebral peduncles(crura cerebri)+Corpora quadrigemina (superior/inf colliculi); Cerebral Aqueduct), **Metencephalon** (Pons+Cerebellum(vermis); Upper 4th ventricle), **Myelencephalon** (Medulla+Pyramids+Olives; Lower 4th ventricle(Magendi/Luschka to subarachnoid space).
5. Cerebral hemispheres – planning of motor activity and perceptual/cognitive functions
6. Frontal lobe: motor, language production, judgement, emotions, memory
7. Parietal lobe: reception/perception of **sensory** from body/emotion/memory
8. Occipital lobe: reception/perception of **visual** information
9. Temporal lobe: reception/perception of **auditory,** visual/emotion/memory
10. Insular lobe: autonomic function – **gustatory**
11. **Thalamus**:transmits/integrates **sensory** info from **Basal ganglia** and **Cerebellum**
12. Thalamus nuclei: VA/VL – to motor cortex, VPL/VPM – to somatosensory cortex, MD – prefrontal cortex, LGeniculateN – to visual cortex, MGN – to auditory cortex, Pulvinar – to posterior association cortex.
13. **Hypothalamus**: homeostasis/reproduction
14. **Midbrain:** transmission of info about **limb** movements, and **eye** movements through auditory and visual info.
15. **Pons:** Ventral: relay motor info Cortex to Cerebellum; Dorsal: respiration/taste/sleep-wake cycle
16. **Cerebellum:** all about posture and balance, thus gets info from **spinal cord**(sensory), **cortex**, **vestibular** apparatus.
17. **Medulla oblongata:** respiration, BP, chemo/mechanosensory info, motor to **neck/face**
18. **Spinal cord**: sensory, motor to body
19. 6 Layers of cerebral cortex:
20. I **Molecular**(plexiform; apical dendrites, few cell bodies),
21. II **External granular layer** (small **inhibitory** interneurons+some pyramidal cell),
22. III **External pyramidal layer** (pyramidal neuron project OUT)**,**
23. IV **Internal granular layer** (interneurons projecting thalamic sensory info to II/III),
24. V **Ganglionic layer**(large pyramidal neurons- major cortical efferents+some corticocortical fibers),
25. VI **Multiform layer**(variety of cells, input from thalamus, II,III,V; axons project to superficial layers and subcortically(thalamus))
26. Golgi (whole neuron), Nissl stain(ER), Weigert stain(myelin)
27. NOTE: Pyramidal cells – output from cortex II,III,V,VI (largest in **V**); Most thalamic sensory neurons end in **IV; cortical association** – mainly in II,III,IV
28. 4 components of **Basal Ganglia:** (Caudate nucleus, [Putamen)$_{striatum}$, Globus pallidus]$_{Lentiform\ nucleus}$, Subthalamic nucleus.
29. **Hippocampus** – process NEW sensory info for memory.

NEUROSCIENCE: The Most Rapid Review Of All Topics

30. Cross-section of Midbrain: **cerebral** peduncles, substantia nigra, medial lemniscus, red nucleus
31. Cross-section of Pons: corticospinal tract, medial lemniscus, **cerebellar** peduncles
32. Cross-section of Medulla: pyramids, olive, medial lemniscus
33. Spinal cord: Cervical(C7/8) and Lumbar(L5) enlargements (limb sensory).
34. Spinal cord: 2 dorsal columns in cervical region – medial column (**gracile fasciculus**) for leg fibers, lateral(**cuneate fasciculus**) for arm.
35. Lateral and Ventral columns of the white matter carry **both** sensory and motor
36. All cranial nerves are Peripheral, BUT CNII (optic)
37. III, IV,VI,XI,XII – NO sensory functions
38. I – **un**myelinated, II- myelinated.
39. V,VII,VIII,IX,X – axons from **peripheral ganglia**
40. EXCEPTION: Sensory from JAW muscle in V: axons from **Mesencephalic nucleus** within CNS
41. III,VII,IX,X – parasympathetic
42. **Corticospinal** tract: Precentral gyrus (**somatotopic**) – corona radiata – Internal capsule – crus cerebri – basilar pons – **PYRAMIDS** (decussation) – lateral corticospinal tract - **contralateral** Ventral horn => Lower Motor neuron
43. **Lobotomy** is substituted with psychoactive drugs.

2. Basic Neuroimaging

1. **Native X-ray** – shows **indirect** sign of brain/spinal pathologies.
2. absorption depends on **density** => 3D onto 2D.
3. **Pneumoencephalography** – to visualize **ventricles** (replace CSF with air)
4. **Cerebral Angiography** – arteries/veins with contract medium- see **arteriovenous malformation, aneurysms**.
5. **Digital Subtraction Angiography** – but can have artefacts if patient moves, see **stenosis, occlusions**.
6. **Myelography** - spinal cord imaging – Contrast medium in subarachnoid space. See **herniated discs**, spinal **tumours**
7. **CAT scan** – see **hemorrhage**, but <u>not acute</u> intracranial infarction.
8. CAT scan with contrast(iodine) is LESS sensitive than MRI for **tumour** diagnosis
9. use CAT scan for ↑intracranial pressure, head trauma – facial/skull fractures
10. Epidural(arterial)/Subdural(venous)/Subarachnoid hemorrhages
11. MRI/MRT/NMR(strong magnetic fields)
12. T1 – **fatty** tissue protons are signal-intense
13. T2 – **water** tissue protons are signal-intense
14. Advantage of MRI- no radiation, can observe Blood Oxygen Level (functional MRI) since deoxyhemoglobin is **paramagnetic**=>observe **active** neurons, BUT can't use with metal(pacemaker)
15. MR Angiography – inject **gadolinium** – paramagnetic medium
16. **Positron Emission Tomography** – use ^{18}F-deoxyglucose(short half life), not metabolized, observe metabolically **active** neurons. Emit **positrons**, which collide with electron and produce 2 γ-rays at 180 degrees.
17. **Single Photon Emission Tomography (SPECT)** – to show **perfusion** in brain, using ^{99m}Tc or ^{123}I, γ-ray cameras for detection.

NEUROSCIENCE: The Most Rapid Review Of All Topics

3. General Morphology

1. **Central** sulcus, **Sylvian** fissure
2. **Parieto-occipital** sulcus(see on median side) and **Preoccipital notch**(on inferior border) make a line that separates parietal and occipital lobes and temporal lobe.
3. **Insular** lobe is surrounded by **circular sulcus.**
4. **Cingulate sulcus** denotes **Limbic lobe**
5. Central sulcus on medial side of brain is the next sulcus anteriorly to **Marginal ramus of Cingulate sulcus.**
6. **Calcarine fissure** (seen on medial side) divides occipital and temporal lobes
7. **Tuber cinereum** – anterior to mammillary bodies, a basis of infundibulum.
8. CN I – telencephalon: olfactory bulb
9. CN II – diencephalons:
10. CN III – brain stem: interpeduncular fossa.
11. CN IV – brain stem: below inferior colliculus
12. CN V – brain stem: pons
13. CN VI – brainstem: pontomedullary junction
14. CN VII – brain stem: pontomedullary junction – closer to middle cerebellar peduncle
15. CN VIII – brain stem: next to VII
16. CN IX – brain stem: **postolivary** sulcus
17. CN X – brain stem: **postolivary** sulcus, next to IX
18. CN XI – brain stem: **postolivary** sulcus, under IX,X,XII
19. CN XII – brain stem: **pre**olivary sulcus
20. Spinal cord: T1-L3 has **intermediolateral cell column**
21. Spinal cord is described by **anterior median fissure, anterolateral sulcus** (ventral root)**, posterolateral sulcus** (dorsal root)**, posterior median sulcus.**
22. conus medullaris (L1-2), cauda equina, filum terminale.
23. Sympathetic chain ganglia: **3c+12t+4l+4s+1cox.**

4. Brain Surface

1. LATERAL:
2. **Frontal lobe**: precentral sulcus, precentral gyrus, superior frontal **gyrus**-superior frontal sulcus-middle frontal gyrus-inferior frontal sulcus-inferior frontal gyrus(pars orbitalis+pars triangularis+pars opercularis[frontal,parietal,temporal parts])
3. **Parietal lobe:** postcentral sulcus, postcentral gyrus, superior parietal **lobule**-intraparietal sulcus-inferior parietal lobule(supramarginal gyrus+angular gyrus)
4. **Temporal lobe:** superior temporal **gyrus**-superior temporal sulcus-middle temporal gyrus-inferior temporal sulcus-inferior temporal gyrus
5. **Occipital lobe:** lunate sulcus, occipital gyri
6. Brodmann map -47-52 areas
7. **Broca**'s speech area: **left** hemisphere- pars triangularis (**45**)+pars opercularis(**44**)
8. **Wernicke's: left** hemisphere- posterior portion of area **22**(temporal lobe) including **planum temporale**
9. Motor cortex – precentral gyrus(**4**).
10. Primary somatosensory cortex- postcentral gyrus (**3,1,2**)
11. **Transverse temporal gyrus of Heschl-** on <u>superior</u> side of temporal lobe (not visible) – primary auditory. Extends into planum temporale and separated from Wernicke's by **transverse temporal sulcus.**
12. **Insular lobe**: most frontal:**limen insulae**, from which short and long gyri radiate, separated by the central sulcus of the insular.
13. INFERIORLY: frontal lobe is separated from parietal by olfactory sulcus, orbital gyri, **gyrus rectus**(continuous with superior frontal gyrus)
14. Olfactory cortex (rhinencephalon): olfactory **bulb/tract,** olfactory **trigone, piriform** cortex, **periamygdaloid** cortex, **entorhinal** cortex.
15. Olfactory trigone: medial olfactory **striae,** lateral olfactory striae, anterior **perforated substance.**
16. MEDIAL:
17. Frontal/parietal lobes: **cingulate** sulcus, para**central** lobule, septum pellucidum(separates anterior horns of lateral ventricles), lamina terminalis
18. Limbic lobe: subcallosal area,cingulate gyrus, parahippocampal gyrus
19. Occipital lobe: calcarine sulcus-cuneus-lingual gyrus
20. Temporal part: uncus-**rhinal** sulcus-parahippocampal g-collateral sulcus-medial occipitotemporal gyrus-occipitotemporal sulcus-lateral occipitotemporal gyrus
21. Corpus callosum:rostrum-genu-body-splenium-sulcus
22. Fornix: bundle of axons from hippocampus to mammillary bodies **under** corpus callosum.
23. **Massa intermedia -** interthalamic adhesion
24. Mesencephalon(midbrain) – posterior tectum (corpora quadrigemini) + anterior tegmentum (floor of midbrain)

5. Meninges and Arteries

1. dural Venous sinus – between two layers of Dura matter
2. Cistern – between pia(vascular) and arachnoid(avascular) matter
3. Subarachnoid hemorrhage (blood in sulci) – **cerebral** arteries between pia and arachnoid matter
4. Intracerebral hemorrhage – hypertensive rupture of intracerebral branch of cerebral artery.
5. Brain meninges (**4**layers) vs Spinal meninges (**3**layers +denticulate ligaments)
6. Cerebral arteries: Internal carotid + Vertebral arteries= circle of Willis & Basilar artery.
7. Internal carotid => **anterior** and **middle** cerebral arteries
8. Vertebral artery=>**posterior** cerebral artery
9. Spinal cord: **2 posterior** spinal arteries (dorsal+lateral) + **1 anterior** (ventral)=anast.
10. Brain: 15% of Cardiac output(1L/min), 20% of Oxygen.
11. **Autoregulation** in cerebral vessels to maintain 60-150mmHg.

6. Ventricles, CSF, Veins, Sinuses

1. Embryonic brain: **Prosencephalon** (telencephalon+diencephalon), **Mesencephalon, Rhombencephalon** (Metencephalon, Myelencephalon)
2. Lateral ventricle: **Anterior horn**(between Corpus callosum(S), septum pellucidum(M), and caudate nucleus(IL)), **Body** (in parietal lobe, posterior to Monro: between splenium Corpus Callosum(PS), Septum pellucidum(M), Inf.:Fornix, choroids plexus, dorsal thalamus, stria terminalis, caudate nucleus), **Inferior horn**(temporal lobe, Medial: fornix/hippocampus/stria terminalis/caudate nucleus, Anterior: Amygdala), **Posterior horn** (occipital lobe: corpus callosum (S), calcarine fissure eminence(M))
3. Third ventricle: ependymal cells(S), Thalami(L), Hypothalamus(I), lamina terminalis/anterior fissure(A)
4. Fourth ventricle: pons/medulla(A), cerebellum/medullary velum(P), cerebellar peduncles(LI); 2xLuschka+Magendie=>subarachnoid space.
5. Choroid plexus: semipermeable filter between blood and CSF in each ventricle, covered with ependyma: floor of lateral ventricle, roof of 3rd, roof of 4th.
6. CSF: protein free, cushion, nutritive and waste removal, with normal pressure 65-200mmH2O(5-15mmHg). **IF find cells**=>meningitis/encephalitis
7. CSF: [Na]=serum, [Cl]>serum, [K,Ca,Mg]<serum
8. CSF: produced@700ml/day from **Choroid** + ependyma/glia/pia-arachnoid cap. beds
9. 140ml – total CSF volume
10. Non-communicating (obstructive) hydrocephalus (block in CSF route – above enlargement) VS Communicating hydrocephalus (↓CSF absorption – all ventricles enlarged)
11. Venous sinuses receive from: **cerebral veins** (great=>superior, small=>transverse, Galen=>straight), **diploic veins**(+meningeal+superficial), **emissary vein**(extracranial+intracranial)
12. KNOW venous sinuses
13. Transverse, Cavernous, and Petrosal sinuses drain to **internal jugular vein**
14. **6** veins around spinal cord (AM, 2AL, 2PL, PM) + Venous Batson.
15. **7** Circumventricular organs – weak BBB=> can be used as blood sensors: **subfornical** organ(thirst), **organum vasculorum**(electrolyte/peptides), **pineal** gland(melatonin), **area postrema** (vomiting centre), **subcommissural** organ (glycoproteins to CSF), **median eminence** (to Ant Pituitary), **neurohypophysis.**
16. Thrombosis of sinuses due to infection in ear, nasopharynx, face,scalp =>HEPARINS

NEUROSCIENCE: The Most Rapid Review Of All Topics

7. Brainstem/Cerebellum

1. **spinal cord**: Alar plate (sensory) is behind the **sulcus limitans**=>dorsal horn, BUT in the **brainstem** Alar plates move laterally=> afferents are lateral (efferents are medial)
2. CHECK for knowledge of brainstem anatomy – p8-4
3. KNOW contents of brainstem (tracts) p8-6
4. **Reticular** formation: **S**- arousal-coordination of licking/chewing/licking/sucking-CV/breathing control-swallowing-vasomotor/expiration-vomiting-inspiration-**I**.
5. **Cerebellar tracts (4):** cerebello-rubral, olivo-cerebellar, Ant/Post spinocerebellar tract
6. **Blood supply** of brainstem: midbrain, pons (basilar), medulla(PICA, AICA, Anterior spinal artery),
7. **Cerebellum**
8. **Wallenberg's syndrome** – occlusion of PICA: loss of sensory ipsilateral in face/contralateral in body, ipsilateral Horner's syndrome, nausea, diplopia, tendency to fall, hoarseness, dysphagia, ataxia.

Module B. Cellular Neuroscience

8. Neurons/Glia

1. Glial cells: **oligodendrocyte, Schwann cell, Astrocyte** (microenvironment), **Microglia**(protect), **Ependymal** cells
2. Glial cells have a membrane potential but do NOT produce Action potential.
3. Neurons: **neurites** – dendrite + axon.
4. Neurons that release **catecholamines/serotonin/peptide** the vesicle is **dense** cored
5. Neurons that release **acetylcholine** (motor neuron) the vesicle is **clear**
6. **Nissl** body – ER's in the neuron cell body – protein production site.
7. Cytoskeleton: **microtubules**(13 protofilaments α->B+, **tau** protein stabilizes), **neurofilaments**(little turnover, scaffold of skeleton, most abundant), **microfilament**(actin, growth cone)
8. **A fibers** – Largest, Fastest
9. **C fibers** – Smallest, Slowest
10. **Afferent fibers-** I, II,... groups of fibers
11. **Kinesin**(~myosin) – anterograde, in + direction, towards nerve ending, on microtubule, move vesicles/mitochondria
12. **Dynein**(~cilia/flagella) – retrograde, in '-' direction, towards soma, on microtubule, move lysosomes, recycled vesicle, **nerve growth factor**.
13. NO **slow** transport by retrograde.
14. Microtubules in dendrites can be directed **either** way.
15. **Astrocyte:** store glycogen/supply Lactate(10min), Remove and distribute(gap junctions, **spatial buffering**) excess K+, Uptake glutamate, glycine, noradrenaline
16. **Ependymal cell:** Group1 (**tight** junctions, secretory, CSF- blood barrier)
17. **Ependymal cell:** Group2 (**GAP** junctions, ciliated, CSF circulation)
18. **Microglia:** =macrophage, phagocytosis
19. **Oligodendrocytes:** myelinate **several** axons in CNS as well as several segments of 1
20. **Schwann cells:** myelinate **single** axon in PNS
21. **Unmyelinated** axons are usually covered in bunch(**Remak fibre**) by non-insulating Schwann (PNS) or Oligodendrocyte+Astrocyte (CNS), which regulates the extracellular K+.
22. !**Schwann cells** facilitate **regeneration** of axons (form a guiding tube and secrete growth factors[**neurotrophins**])
23. **Wallerian** – anterograde, distal degeneration of cut axon
24. **Oligodendrocytes** – do **NOT** form guiding tubes and secrete very little growth factor
25. GLIOSIS – hyper**plasia** and hyper**trophy** of **astrocytes** in neuronal injury in CNS, that leaves **scars**.
26. GLIAL tumours – 50% of brain, 25% of spinal tumours
27. NEURONAL tumours – RARE
28. VIRUS (herpes, rabies) – use **retrograde** transport to get to cell body and destroy it.

NEUROSCIENCE: The Most Rapid Review Of All Topics

9. Resting Excitable cells.

1. Very **little** of an ion required to cross the membrane to change Vm **significantly**.
2. Cations move to Cathode(-), Anions move to Anode(+)
3. Open channel speed: 10^7 ions/sec
4. ATPases (10^3): Ca, H, Na_3/K_2
5. Neurotransmitters: Symport(Na+) to nerve terminals, Antiport(H+) to synaptic vesicles.
6. Depolarization (add Cations **outside**) VS Hyperpolarization (add Cations **inside**)
7. Neuron: K+channels open frequently VS Skeletal muscle:K+,Cl- open frequently
8. Voltage-gated(Po depends on **Vm**) VS Ligand-gated(Po depends on **Concentration**)
9. Channels **open**=Po x Total channels
10. **Single** Channel conductance (inverse of resistance) ~10pSiemens
11. **Nernst equation:** Ex= 61/z x Log Xo/Xi mV @ **37C°**
12. In both skeletal and neurons only **Cl-** ions are close to equilibrium at **rest;** ie E_{Cl}=Em
13. **Electrochemical gradient** – how far the Em is from equilibrium (ie Driving force)
14. Membrane=Equivalent Circuit of **Capacitors**(bilipid layer) and **Resistors** (channels)
15. Total **C** and **R** are both calculated by simple addition of individual units.
16. NET current at REST is ZERO (Na_{in}, K_{out}, Cl)
17. Vm is the **Weighted sum** of the Equilibrium Potentials of ions (Course grade analogy)
18. LETHAL INJECTION: K+Cl- solution=> depolarization, tissues non-excitable(↓heart)
19. Ischaemic Cerebral Edema – **cytotoxic edema** due to Na entry into cells because of failed Na/K ATPase; followed by **vasogenic edema** (vessels become permeable)

10. Stimulated Excitable Cells

1. Mechanoreceptors, Photoreceptors(cones/rods), Chemoreceptors(olfactory)
2. *Change of conductance is **NOT** spread to adjacent regions, change of Vm **IS**.
3. **Local** graded potential is spread with **decrement**
4. **Length constant** - how far from stimulation site will the Vm become 37% (1/e) of original graded potential. **(V=Vo exp(-x/lambda))**
5. **Lambda α Radius, Resistance**
6. Muscle mechanoreceptors(Ia)–**Muscle spindle** (length) &**Golgi tendon organ**(tension)
7. **Intrafusal fibers** in muscle are **non-contractile,** contain mechanoreceptors with stretch-gated **Na** channels
8. **Graded potential,** ie depends on the strength of the stimulus: ex **Ia**: stretchαVm
9. **Rods:** rhodopsin absorbs photons, that activate G protein, which activates **Phosphodiesterase,** which **breaks down cGMP.** cGMP keeps Na channel open =>depolarized membrane @-40mV. So, ↓cGMP=>↓Na channels open =>**hyperpolarization.** Since response to light depends on intensity of light – the hyperpolarization is **graded.**, which spreads to rod's nerve ending and ↓transmitter release onto bipolar cells of retina.
10. **NOTE: graded** responses of membranes to stimuli **may or may not** cause Action Potential. Depends if the **depolarizing** graded potential reaches the **threshold**. Once the threshold is reached and AP fires, any **larger** stimuli will **NOT** produce **greater** effect.
11. **NOTE: hyperpolarizing** graded potentials do not induce Action Potential
12. **Olfactory:** bipolar neurons bind odorant chemicals and G protein activates **Adenylate Cyclase,** which produces **cAMP.** This leads to **protein kinases'** activation and **phosphorylation** of cation(Na, Cl) channel to **open** state. Depolarization also causes **Cl channels** to open, which further contribute to depolarization ([Cl]i=80mM!=> E_{Cl}=-15mv=> outward Cl gradient at Vm). The response is again **GRADED,** and depends on odorant concentration.
13. **Initiation zone (↑Na channel [])** – can be at axon hillock(multipolar motor n.), endings(sensory n), or central(**muscle @NMJ**)
14. p11-12 AP(all-or-none) vs Graded Potential(αstimuli)
15. ANOSMIA – loss of olfactory
16. NIGHT BLINDNESS - ↓VitA=>↓Rhodopsin in rods.

11. AP Initiation & Conduction

1. **Threshold:** Na influx **exceeds** K efflux. =>more depolarization=>↑Na channel open
2. Depolarization also activates voltage-gated K channels BUT with a delay.
3. At AP's peak Na influx=K efflux (g_{Na} x (Vm-E_{Na})) = g_K x (Vm-E_K)
4. **Inactivation** of Na channel – depolarization induced (↓g_{Na})
5. **Voltage-gated channel:** 4 subunits/6 TM segments each, Segment 4 is **charged** (voltage-sensor), Each subunit has a **pore loop**(ion selectivity).
6. **Ball and chain** model: inactivating subunit(+ charge) blocks the pore of Na channel from inside in depolarization => contribute to **absolute refractory period**
7. **Relative** refractory period: some Na channel are in **normal** closed state(not inactivated), and can be opened by a large stimulus BUT in this period lots of K channels are still open and oppose Na influx.
8. Na,K channel distribution: **un**myelinated axons/skeletal muscle (uniform-100/microm^2), myelinated axons (Na channels –high@nodes of **Ranvier**-2000/microm^2, K-channels – high **paranodal** 800/microm^2).
9. **Nodal impulse:** NO hyperpolarization, since there is NO K channels at nodes.
10. **Demyelination** of myelinated axon impairs conduction due to large spread of V-gated Na channels
11. **AP – continuous conduction** without decrement (positive charge propagates **internally** in both myelinated and unmyelinated)
12. **Saltatory conduction:** in myelinated axon, the Length Constant is large. (note: there is also a backward move of positive charge **extracellularly** from inactive node to active)
13. Speed of conduction α fiber **diameter** (fiber+myelin): m/s = **6** x micr**o**m
14. Myelination: ↑velocity, saves space (can have smaller diameter fibers), saves energy (localized ATPases)
15. TETRODOTOXIN (marine bacteria) / SAXITOXIN (marine dinoflagellates) – block Na-channels from **OUTSIDE**
16. LIDOCAINE/PROCAINE block Na-channels from **INSIDE,** Adelta(small unmyelinated)>C fibers (unmyelinated)> large myelinated axons.
17. **A**delta & **C** fibers – pain transmitters
18. **Demyelination** reduces the **safety factor** (current at active node is **5x** of necessary to initiate AP at the next node) by loss of +ve charge across internodal membrane of axon
19. **Demyelination: Frequency-related block** (some AP are not transmitted to the next node through the unmyelinated region), **Total Conduction Block, "Crosstalk"** between unmyelinated axons.
20. MULTIPLE SCLEROSIS – **autoimmune** against **Oligodendrocytes;** among others, CN II is the ONLY cranial nerve that's demyelinated.
21. GUILLAIN-BARRE syndrome: **autoimmune** against **Schwann;** ascending paralysis

12. Synaptic Transmission in Spinal Cord

1. 2 types of synapses: **electrical**(GAP junction: ex. Pyramidal cells in hippocampus, retina horizontal cells, astrocytes) and **chemical**(boutons with vesicles at **active zone**
2. **Axosomatic** synapses: mostly **inhibitory** on postsynaptic neuron **firing rate**
3. **Axodendritic** synapses: mostly **excitatory** on postsynaptic neuron **firing rate**
4. **Axoaxonic** synapse: mostly **inhibitory** on postsynaptic neurotransmitter **release**
5. Synaptic delay always present: 0.5ms-100ms
6. 2 types of transmitter **receptors**: **Ionotropic** (ion channels) + **Metabotropic**(G-p.C.R.)
7. 3 mechanisms for transmitter **removal**: **Diffusion**(neuropeptides), EC Enzymatic **Degradation**(ACh), **Uptake** to nerve endings/glia(catecholamines, serotonin, glutamate) where it's broken down.
8. **Myotatic reflex** – sensory from muscle(Ia) synapses5x(**Glutamate**) on each of 100s of motors neuron for that muscle. + Ia also synapse on **inhibitory interneurons** that synapses(**Glycine**) on antagonist muscle (aka **Reciprocal Innervation**)
9. **Glutamate** activates **AMPA** receptor (E_{Na+K}= -0.85mV; Na, K channel, $I_{Na}>I_K$=>depolarization), causing $E_{xcitotory}P_{ost}S_{ynaptic}P_{otential}$ (~1mV change from one channel), which has a rapid depolarizing phase and slow repolarizing phase(tau constant).
10. Amplitude of EPSP depends on Glutamate concentration.
11. AMPA **Reversal Potential** (NO **synaptic** flow) ~ E_{Na+K}= -0.85mV
12. **Glycine**(from inhibitory interneuron) activates ionotropic receptor (E_{Cl}= -65mV; Cl channel) causing $I_{nhibitory}PSP$, which moves Em towards E_{Cl}(up or down) and has a rapid falling phase and slow repolarizing phase. Again, the **reversal potential** for the channel is E_{Cl}.
13. **Threshold:** NOT a set value; it is a Em at which inward Na current(depends on the number of Na channels) is starts to outweigh the outward K current (depends on the number of K channels)=> threshold varies with channel **densities**
14. The more Na channels, the lower the threshold, the more excitable is the membrane, hence:
15. **Motor** neurons: Highest Na channel concentration is at the **axon hillock**=>most excitable at the hillock (**initiation zone**)
16. **Sensory** neurons: Highest Na channel concentration is at the sensory **ending** (NOT hillock)
17. **EPSP's** spread with Decrement from synapse to **initiation zone**
18. **Spatial** summation: EPSPs from different synapses arriving to same initiation zone cause **additive** effect.
19. **Temporal** summation: because repolarizing phase of EPSP is slow(see point 9), the **next** EPSP in the same region will **add** to depolarization.
20. Both EPSPs and IPSPs can add both spatially and temporally.
21. TETANUS TOXIN: from bacillus through skin, by **retrograde** axonal transport to cell bodies of **ventral roots**, then to inhibitory interneuron and ↓Glycine release=>hyperreflexia, spasms.
22. STRYCHNINE poisoning: plant alkaloid, blocks CNS Glycine receptor=> spasms, convulsions, ↓breathing
23. COCAINE: blocks **reuptake** of dopamine, noradrenaline, serotonin.
24. MORPHINE: like **mu-enkephalin**(from inhibitory neurons), binds to C fiber(pain) terminals(in Substantia gelatinosa of dorsal horn) and inhibit transmitter(SubstanceP/glutamate) release => pain is not relayed to second order neurons in spinal cord.

NEUROSCIENCE: The Most Rapid Review Of All Topics

13. Neuromuscular Transmission

1. Motor unit= cell body+axon+(**non-myelin,Schwann covered**)NMJ(ACh to **end plate**)+muscle fiber
2. The number of muscle fibers innervated by one neuron depends on how **fine** the control of movement required
3. There is NO inhibitory synapses on **muscle fibers**
4. ACh is made by **Choline Acetyltransferase**(good marker for cholinergic neurons) in cytosol of **cholinergic** nerve terminals ONLY
5. ACh is broken down by **Acetylcholinesterase**(NOT good marker) in the **cleft** of synapse and the **choline** is reuptaken by **Na-Choline symporter**
6. ACh binds **ionotropic(Nicotinic) and metabotropic(Muscarinic)**
7. ACh exocytosis is initiated by Ca influx through voltage-gated Ca channel upon AP
8. ACh at the **end plate** on ACh-gated channels causes depolarization, which activates **Voltage-gated Na channels** in the junctional folds and initiates AP across muscle fiber
9. Ionotropic ACh-gated receptor: 5 subunits: $2\alpha,B,\gamma,delta$. EACH α binds 1Ach.
10. **Fetal** nAChR: $2\alpha,B,\gamma,delta$; smaller currents, longer mean open time
11. **Adult** nAChR: $2\alpha,B,$**Theta**,delta: larger currents, more frequent but short open times
12. Ionotropic ACh-gated receptor: Needs BOTH ACh to **open**, further – **desensitization.**
13. Ionotropic ACh-gated receptor: Cause $E_{nd}P_{late}P_{otential}$ that spread with decrement. However(!), unlike neuronal synapse, **1 AP from the nerve** produces enough depolarization(T tubule=>↑Ca from SR) at the end plate to cause a **muscle fiber twitch.**
14. Toxins on Motor Unit: **V-gated Na channels**: TETRODOTOXIN, SAXITOXIN
15. Toxins on Motor Unit: ↓ACh release: BOTULINUM(blocks vesicle docking=>flaccid paralysis), α-LATROTOXIN(initial ACh release(contraction) followed by NO more(flaccid paralysis)), omega-CONOTOXIN(Irreversible binding of V-gated Ca channels=>↓ACh release=>flaccid paralysis)
16. Toxins on Motor Unit: ↓**Acetylcholinesterase:** PHYSOSTIGMINE, NEOSTIGMINE, Malathion/Parathion(Irreversible), NERVE GAS(sarin, tabun) =>death due to respiratory paralysis.
17. Toxins on Motor Unit: ↑**nAChR:** CARBACHOL, NICOTINE, SUCCINYLCHOLINE(aka suxamethonium) - all **agonists,** none degraded by AChE
18. Toxins on Motor Unit: ↓**nAChR:** TUBOCURARINE(reversible), PANCURONIUM(rev), α-BUNGAROTOXIN(irrev) - all **antagonists,** flaccid paral.
19. HEXAMETHONIUM: ACh antagonist at synapse in Sympathetic ganglia
20. LAMBERT-EATON syndrome: autoimmune disease against **V-gated Ca-channels**=>bad conduction. 4-AMINOPYRIDINE – blocks **K channel** to prolong depolarization=>↑Ca entry at boutons. NEOSTIGMINE – ↓ACh breakdown.
21. MYASTHENIA GRAVIS: autoimmune disease against **nAChR**=>bad conduction. Treat with NEOSTIGMINE to ↓ACh breakdown + ATROPINE(ACh antagonist in Cardiovascular system)
22. Anesthesia: Depolarizing agents(nAChR agonists, keep Na-channel inactive=>inexcitable): Succinylcholine - fast but **short** effects
23. Anesthesia: Non-Depolarizing agents(nACh antagonists): Curare/Pancuronium -long-acting

14. Transmitter release

1. Vesicles store **Small-molecule transmitter**(made in cytosol of nerve ending, stored in **Clear** vesicle(~10000) <u>closer</u> to **active zones**: ACh, Glutamate)and **Neuropeptide**(made in soma to **Large dense core** vesicle, anterograde transport: Peptides+NE/Serotonin)
2. Transmitter transport into vesicle α on H+ gradient (H ATPase):**Dopamine-H antiport**
3. Exocytosis(**p x n**): tethering of vesicle to cytoskeleton (**synapsin**), trafficking to exocytosis site(**Rab**), docking/priming with nerve membrane (**synaptobrevin/synaptotagmin**), fusion with nerve membrane (**synaptophysin**)
4. AP reaches terminal=> Ca influx(**fast**)=>Phosphorylation of synapsin(untethering) by **Ca-calmodulin-dependent PK** and vesicle release. Ca is **extruded**(Ca ATPase/ Ca/Na exchange) and **stored** in sER:**slow**
5. Docking by $v_{esicular}$-**SNAREs** and $t_{erminal}$-*SNAREs*: **synaptobrevin**+*syntaxin*; **synaptotagmin**+*neurexin*
6. 10Hz =>↑Ca close to **active zone: Clear** vesicle release
7. 100Hz=>↑Ca further from **active zone: Dense core** vesicle release
8. NT's (NOT ACh) are taken up**rapid**)to nerve terminals(or glial):Glycine, NA, glutamate
9. Endocytosis recycles membrane and uptakes extracellular material (NOT NT's) by **clathrin**-coating: Clear vesicle membrane->**Endosome**;
    Dense core vesicle membrane->**Soma** by **retrograde**(dynein on MT)
10. Spontaneous ACh release causes $min_{iature}E_{nd}P_{late}P_{otential}$ – **quantum**
11. Quantal hypothesis: AP-> n x vesicle released, n=0,1,2,3..
12. BOTULINUM: irreversibly breaks down synaptobrevin(docking)=.↓ACh release (double vision, ↓swallowing, dry mouth, ↓speaking, limb weakness, **respiratory**);use in **dystonia, cosmetic surgery**(↓facial wrinkle)
13. TETANUS: retrograde to CNS, interneurons' synaptobrevin↓=>↓Glycine (spasms)
14. α-LATROTOXIN: binds *neurexin*/**synaptotagmin** complex=>↑exocytosis=>depletes ACh (smasm-flaccid cycles)
15. NEOMYCIN>STREPTOMYCIN: inhibit ACh exocytosis. Reverse by ↑Ca
16. Axo-axonic synapses with GABA, serotonin, dopamine=>↓exocytosis
17. hypo**para**thyroidism=>HYPOCALCEMIA=> ↑-ve sialic acid (carbs) around membrane~depolarization AND ↑leakeness of membrane=>more excitable=>**tetany** and **paresthesias**

15. Neurotransmitter systems

1. 4 types of Neurotransmitters: amino acids(fast), amines(fast), peptides, gases(NO to intracellular **Guanylate cyclase=>↑cGMP**
2. NA on α (+phenylephrine, -phenoxybenzamine); on Beta(+Isoproterenol,-Propranolol)
3. Glutamate on AMPA(+AMPA, -CNQX); on NMDA(+NMDA, -AP5)
4. GABA on A(+muscimol, -bicuculline); on B(+baclofen, -phaclofen)
5. Glycine R(+glycine, -strychnine)
6. Serotonin is reabsorbed and deaminated by $M_{ono}A_{mine}O_{xidase}$.
7. NA is reabsorbed, deaminated by MAO; methylated(catechol) by $C_{atechol}O M_{ethyl}T_{ransferase}$
8. **Muscarinic** R's:M1/M3 (slow excitatory;salivary/lacrimal1 & gastric acid/**contraction** of smooth muscles3), M2(inhibitory)
9. **M1/M3=>**G-pcr=>↑PLC=>↑IP3/DAG=>↑Ca from sER=>↑product secretion.
10. M2(cardiac pacemaker under PNS)=>G_i-pcr=>↓AC=>↓cAMP=>↓Ca channels =>↓contr
    (Shortcut pathway) G_i-pcr=>↑K channel=>↓contractility of heart
11. Catecholaminergic neurons: tyrosine[**tyrosine hydroxylase**]DOPA[**dopa decarboxylase***]Dopamine[**dopamine B-hydroxylase** (vesicles ONLY)]NA/$A_{chromaffin}$
12. **Beta1** receptor(cardiac pacemaker): Gs-pcr=>↑AC=>↑cAMP=>↑gCa, ↓gK=>↑f and F.
13. **Glycine R** : 3α2Beta – Cl channel
14. $GABA_A$ - **2α2Beta1γ** - **ionotropic** – fast, inhibitory; **benzodiazepines+** on α, **barbiturates+** on γ.
15. $GABA_B$ – **metabotropic** – slow inhibitory---➔↑K channel open
16. Glutamate on AMPA(Na) and NMDA(Ca). NMDA is blocked by Mg, which is release at **large** depolarization due to EPSPs summation
17. BRAIN: Cholinergic neurons (septal nucleus, n.ofMeynett, pons) – **ascending arousal system** - ↑arousal in wake and REM
18. BRAIN: Noradrenergic neurons (**locus coeruleus**➔hippocampus, amygdala, hypothalamus, thalamus, cerebellum, cortex) - **ascending arousal system, MOOD**
19. BRAIN: Serotonergic neurons (**rostral raphe n.**➔hippocampus, amygdala, hypothalamus, thalamus, cortex) - **ascending arousal system, MOOD**
20. BRAIN: Serotonergic neurons (**caudal raphe n.**➔dorsal horn) – **nociception**
21. BRAIN: Dopamine ($D_{1,5}$-↑cAMP; $D_{2,3,4}$-↓cAMP) (**substantia nigra**(Parkinson)➔basal ganglia (caudate n+putamen, BOTH D1 and D2) (**ventral tegmental area**➔hippocampus, nucleus accumbens, frontal lobe cortex)
22. D2 agonists for Parkinson, D2 antagonists for psychotic conditions
23. Opioid peptides (YGGF, ex **enkephalin, morphine**) on 3 types of R's: mu, delta, kappa
24. Amygdala: fear and anxiety, has GABAa R
25. $S_{elective}S_{erotonin}R_{euptake}I_{nhibitor}$s (fluoxetine) for depression treatment (better that MAO inhibitors)
26. PILOCARPINE ~ACh, for ↑fluid drainage=>↓intraocular pressure (pressure)
27. Beta blockers (PROPRANOLOL) for Hypertension
28. Beta2 agonist (SALBUTAMOL) for ↓asthmatic bronchoconstriction
29. Alpha1 agonist (PHENYLEPHRINE) ↓vasoconstriction in nose=>↓nasal congestion

Timur M. Urakov

NEUROSCIENCE: The Most Rapid Review Of All Topics

16. Transport within CNS

1. Normal Intracranial Pressure = 65-200 mmWater (5-15mmHg), but spinal tap is unreliable if there is an obstruction.
2. CSF vs plasma: **less** protein, Glu, K, Ca=>↓pH; **more** Cl, Mg; **same** Osm, Na, ~HCO3
3. CSF (4): maintains environ, route of metabolite removal, pH changes affect Respiration/cerebral blood flow, mechanical cushion
4. BBB: tight junctions between cell do not allow **paracellular route**(between cells), lipid soluble molecules must go through the endothelial cells (**Transcellular route**)
5. ?Glucose/L-dopa do not lie on expected transport rate line (sigmoid), due to facilitation
6. Glucose **faster** than expected due to GLUT1 transporter (facilitated diffusion)
7. Glycine crosses BBB by secondary active transport with Na.
8. BBB ↑ leakiness by(4): Hypertension, Hyperosmolarity(shrinks cells), Infection, Trauma(ischemia, inflammation, pressure)
9. Ventricles are lined by Ependymal cells Group1(+beating cilia) and Group2(secretory choroids plexus) with Blood-CSF barrier:
10. The blood-CSF barrier epithelial cells have channels for Na, K, Cl, Na/K ATPase and specifically: **Apical** membrane(microvilli): K, Cl cotransporter; **Basolateral** membrane:Na/K/Cl cotransporters=> net Na, Cl, K into the ventricle + water = 500ml/day
11. **CSF** is reabsorbed in **Superior Sagittal Sinus** through **arachnoid villi** due to pressure, via **transcellular vacuoles**
12. CSF for diagnostic: <5 cells/cm3+35 mg/dlProtein+60mg/dlGlucose = NORMAL
13. CSF for diagnostic: ↑lymphocytes+↑protein=**Viral** meningitis/Brain tumour
14. CSF for diagnostic: ↑Neutrophils+↑protein+↓Glucose= **Bacterial** meningitis
15. CSF for diagnostic: ↑IgG = **Multiple Sclerosis**
16. CSF for diagnostic: <10Leukocytes +↑protein= **Guillain-Barre syndrome**
17. CSF for diagnostic: ↑RBS+↑protein = **Subarachnoid** hemorrhage
18. **Hydrocephalus**: Non-communicating(Obstructive), Communicating(↓Absorption=>**All** ventricles enlarge)
19. **Normal Pressure Hydrocephalus** – due to aging.
20. **Monro-Kellie doctrine:** When a mass lesion increase one CSF compartment, there will be an increase in pressure (ICP) unless another compartment is reduced.
21. **Cerebral perfusion pressure**= Arterial pressure – ICP
22. **Edema: Vasogenic(**damage to capillaries(**white** matter)=>more permeable to plasma proteins: brain tumour, abscess, trauma, hemorrhage)
23. **Edema: Cytotoxic(**hypoxia/ischemia/toxins=>↓ATPase=>ionic gradient dissipates=>cells **swell** = damage in **grey&white** matter, BUT permeability is normal.
24. Tumours in CNS(astrocytoma/glioblastoma) supplied by non BBB capillaries =>↑nutrients paracellularly
25. Dandy-Walker Syndrome: foramen of Luschka/Magendie fail to develop.

Module C. Development

17. Nervous System Development

1. Neuroembryology: Initially all cells in embryo are electrically coupled. $B_{one}M_{orphgenic}P_{rotein}$ stimulates **neural plate** cell formation from ectoderm(uncoupling). Neural **tube** forms due to **change in cell shape**, NOT due to division. **Folic acid** helps in tube folding.
2. Segmentation: 1st: **Homeobox**(conserved) genes – TF's. Facilitate Rhombencephalon (hindbrain) segmentation (ex: kreisler, Krox-20, Eph). **Hox** genes(~homeotic regulator of Drosophila) act **within** segments. **Retinoic acid** from Hensen's node creates a gradient over embryo that determines the **Hox Ant-Post** pattern in Hindbrain.
3. Segmentation: 2nd:**Sonic Hedgehog (Dorsal-Ventral axis)** from Notochord to induce **floor plate** formation and motorneurons, as well as anterior hindbrain(serotonergic), anterior midbrain (oculomotor neurons), and posterior midbrain (dopaminergic)
4. Cell Proliferation: nuclei of cells in neural tube migrate from ventricular to pial and back surfaces as cell divide. Neurons do not divide and migrate along **radial glia** (Muller in retina, Bergman in cerebellum). **All** neurons form before birth (EXCEPT: granule cells in cerebellum, **Olfactory** neurons(also regenerate))
5. Cell Migration: **on radial glial** cells that extend from ventricular to pial surfaces. Migration mediated by **astrotactin** and **integrin**(ECM adhesion molecule Receptor). **Reelin** – signals when to get 'off' the glial monorail (Reeler mice: Cajal-Retzius cell in marginal cortex). Position of central neurons does NOT affect its predetermined function.
6. Cell Migration: **without radial glial** cells: **GnRH** neurons migrate from olfactory pit into CNS hypothalamus (Kallmann's syndrome olfactory placode malformation=>↓sex mature). **Neural crest** cells migrate along **laminin** and others of ECM.
7. Cell Maturation/Commitment: Identity of peripheral nerves CAN be determined by the **local** environment ($L_{eukemia}I_{nhibitory}F_{actor}$ causes cholinergic commitment and immune differentiation).
8. Cell Maturation/Commitment: Axon growth is due to **diffusible molecules**(filapodia: ex axons of developing spinal cord attracted to **netrin; 'pioneer'** axons(large extensive filapodia) lead the way) and **ECM molecules (laminin** from Schwann cell after injury).
9. Cell Maturation/Commitment: **Myelin** formation depends on **PMP-22**(peripheral myelin protein). Ex 'Trembler' mouse, Charcot-Marie-Tooth disease(Gly->Asp)
10. Cell Maturation/Commitment: **Fasciculation** of fibers is influenced by **N-CAMs** (neural cell adhesion molecules)
11. Cell Maturation/Commitment: there is specific matching between neurons and their targets. Ex: ACh R on muscle are **spread** before the innervation and **concentrated** after by **Agrin** protein, which also plays a role in axon guiding after injury.
12. Cell Survival/Death: **Nerve Growth Factor** found in animal Salivary glands.
13. Cell Survival/Death: **Sympathetics** and other PeripheralNS cell types require NGF at specific time in development
14. Cell Survival/Death:**NGF** enhances neurite outgrowth, and ensures survival of the nerve cell
15. Cell Survival/Death:NGF is uptaken by nerve terminals and transport by **retrograde system** to soma.
16. Cell Survival/Death: Brain-derived neurotrophic factor (**BDNF**) needed for connections in CNS. (NGF+BDNF+NT3,4/5,6 –**neurotrophin family**)
17. Early in development **neurons** produce neutrophils; later in development **target tissues**

18. Cell Survival/Death: There are 2 type of NGF receptors: low affinity, fast- p75(cell death?), and high affinity R's: **TrkA** (NGF), **TrkB** (BDNF, NT4/5), **TrkC** (NT3). High affinity receptors have EC NT-binding domain and IC – Tyr Kinase =>↑PLC, PI-3Kinase, MAP Kinase pathways.
19. Cell Survival/Death: experiments showed importance of NGF for hippocampal cholinergic neurons, BDNF for retinal ganglion cells, cortical neurons, visual cortex.
20. Cell Survival/Death: halfway through development, many growing neurons die – outcompeted for growth factors.
21. Specificity of Connection: at first skeletal muscles are **polyneuronally innervated**, followed by synapse retraction.
22. Specificity of Connection: by **repulsive interaction** between **ephrin** (concentration highest in **posterior** visual tectum) and **ephrin-Receptor** on growing axons(High [R] in Nasal ganglion axons)=>nasal ganglion synapse in Anterior; temporal ganglia(fewer Receptors) in Posterior.
23. Specificity of Connection: Ocular dominance columns establish pattern in layer IVc according to **experience during critical period** in childhood=>congenital squint/astigmatism must be fixed early before the pattern is established ← There are similar patterns for auditory and olfactory systems development.
24. Regeneration and Repair: muscle cell ↑ACh Receptors after denervation and induce axon growth and new synapse formation. In CNS, proteins from astrocytes/oligodendroglia inhibit axon growth but can help with embryonic neuron grafts.
25. Developmental defects: THALIDOMIDE: primary effect on neurons, secondary effect on bone growth; ALBINISM: also exhibit 'miswiring' or **retinogeniculate connections**. Cascading effect of genetic defects, since molecules used at different stages.

Module D. Sensory Systems.

18. Sensory systems. Overview.

1. **4** receptors for all sensory systems: Mechano-, Thermo-, Chemo-, Photo-receptors
2. **3** components of Sensory receptor: Receptor potential(graded), Action Potential(trigger zone, axon), Transmitter release.
3. Sensory receptors: receptors neurons & receptor cells(hair cells in Golgi apparatus – no axon)
4. **4** stimulus attributes – **modality**(type of stimulus, 'labeled line code'), **Intensity**(Frequency code & Population code), **Duration**(slowly adapting receptors(monitor constant stimulation(physiological)), rapidly adapting receptors(monitor changes)), **Location**(where **stimulus** originated- **receptive field** of neuron)
5. **3** basic wiring mechanisms of NS: **Convergence**(2nd order neurons receive from many 1st order neurons), **Divergence**, **Lateral Inhibition**(1st order, Interneurons, 2nd order neurons)

19. Somatosensory System

1. 5 modalities: **Touch**(Merkel's disk(discriminative touch), Ruffini's endings(stretch)), **Vibration**(Meissner's corpuscle(50Hz), Pacinian corpuscle(300Hz)), **Pain**(rapid/slow adapting)/**Temperature**(cold/warm R)(free nerve endings), **Proprioception**(muscle spindle(**Ia**-rapidly adapting to **stretch, II**-slowly adapting to **length**), Golgi tendon organs(**Ib**- reverse myotatic reflex) through **pseudo-unipolar n**
2. **Cutaneous Receptors:** have **adaptation rates**(fast-Meissner/Pacinian; slow-Merkel, Ruffini)/**receptive field sizes**(smaller at surface-Merkel's, Meissner's; larger deeper-Pacinian, Ruffini's).
3. **Fiber types:** myelinated Large/Medium(120m/s, cutaneous mechanoreceptors/proprioceptors), Small(5m/s)/Unmyelinated(<2m/s)(pain and temperature)
4. **Dermatomes-** segmental organization of spinal nerves. with **overlaps**. (C2,C6,C7,C8,T4,T10,L1,L5,S1)
5. Touch/Vibration/Proprioception carried by **Dorsal Column-Medial Lemniscus** with neurons from higher regions of the body being more lateral within the Dorsal Column (Leg fibers in **gracile fasciculus**(medial) synapse in **gracile nucleus** of medulla; Arm fibers in **cuneate fasciculus** synapse **cuneate nucleus** of medulla)
6. Pain/Temperature afferent fibers synapse in **dorsal column,** postsynaptic axons cross to **contralateral Anterolateral System**(Spinothalamic) (NOTE: 2nd order fibers from Leg are lateral in Anterolateral system; Fibers from arm – medial)
7. **Lissauer's Tract:** Not all postsynaptic fibers in Anterolateral system originate from the same spinal level where the sensory enters. Collaterals of some sensory afferents(1st order) before entering the dorsal horn may travel up or down in **dorsolateral fasciculus** (zone of Lissauer) and synapse at different level.
8. SHINGLES(herpes zoster): after chickenpox, herpes virus is in DRG – dermatome affected
9. BROWN-SEQUARD SYNDROME – **hemisection** of the spinal cord – dissociated sensory loss pattern- key for now is that pain/temp sensation is NOT lost in lesions proximity because of Lissauer's tract of collaterals.
10. SYRINGOMYELIA – enlarged **central** canal disrupts cross of 2nd order pain/temp fiber through **anterior white fissure** to Anterolateral system

20. Touch

1. **Body Touch Route:** receptor-1ˢᵗ order neuron-dorsal column-nucleus in lower medulla(cuneate/gracile)-2ⁿᵈ order neuron CROSS to contralateral **medial lemniscus- ventral posteroLateral nucleus** of Thalamus-3ʳᵈ order fibers-**posterior limb of internal capsule** – corona radiata – **S1(primary somatosensory cortex).**
2. **Trigeminal nerve Touch Route:** 1st order neuron- **Principal (chief) sensory nucleus of CN V** in **upper half of Pons**- 2ⁿᵈ order neuron CROSS to contralateral **Ventral trigeminothalamic tract- ventral posterior Medial nucleus-** 3ʳᵈ order neurons- **genu of internal capsule-corona radiata – S1**
3. Primary Somatosensory Cortex: **Topographical organization**(somatotopic map), **Organization in columns**(Slowly/Fast Adapting receptors have separate columns), **Input Layer 4**(1_{pia}-$6_{white\ matter}$, thalamo-cortical fibers synapse in **4**)
4. Two point discrimination α density of touch fibers: high density(low threshold) at finger tip(↑Merkel/Meissner, ↓Ruffini/Pacinian), Low density/High threshold at upper arm, thigh.
5. **4 factors** affecting Spatial Resolution: **density** of cutaneous mechanoreceptors, **small receptive fields** of Merkel/Meissner's, **larger cortical area** involved, **lateral inhibition** ↑resolution.
6. Neurological examination: **Touch**(sharp/dull), **Vibration**(tuning fork), **Proprioception**(toe up/down?), **Two point discrimination** (one or two?), **Stereognosis** (what is it?), **Graphesthesia** (what letter was drawn?).
7. TABES DORSALIS – syphilis => DRG destruction=>↓Large axons(touch/proprioception) but Pain/Temp sensation is OK.
8. PHANTOM LIMB Sensation: cortical area from amputated limb is overtaken by other sensory areas – ie **reorganization of cortical maps.**

21. PAIN

1. two types: Nociceptive (from activated receptor), Neuropathic (aberrant processing in NS)
2. **First pain** (sharp, myelinated A-delta fibers – fast) vs **Second pain** (burning, **un**myelinated C fibers – slower)
3. Pain receptors – NONE in Brain, but present in meninges
4. Visceral/deep Pain – transmitted by unmyelinated **C-fibers** ~ **Referred pain** as cutaneous.
5. **Body Pain Route:** receptor-1st order neuron-synapse in dorsal column (**substantia gelatinosa**)- 2nd order neuron CROSS to contralateral AnteroLateral System- **ventral posteroLateral nucleus** of Thalamus-3rd order fibers-**posterior limb of internal capsule – corona radiata – S1(primary somatosensory cortex).**
6. **Trigeminal nerve Pain Route:** 1st order neuron- enter at Pons and **descend to lower 3rd of spinal nucleus of CN 5 (lower medulla)**- 2nd order neuron CROSS to contralateral **Ventral trigeminothalamic tract- ventral posterior Medial nucleus** of Thalamus- 3rd order neurons- **genu of internal capsule-corona radiata – S1**
7. types of Nociceptors: mechanical (high threshold), thermal, chemical(K^+(damaged cell), Bradykinin(blood), Histamines(mast cells)).
8. Tissue damage=> ↑Prostaglandins, Leukotrienes, Substance P=> **sensitization of nociceptors => hyperalgesia.**
9. **Regulation of Pain:** Afferent and Descending
10. Afferent regulation of pain: Touch fibers (large myelinated) activate **inhibitory interneurons** within the dorsal **horn,** which use **enkephalin** to stimulate **opioid receptors** on afferent neurons(↓**AP duration**), presynaptic ending(↓**EPSP**), and postsynaptic site(**hyperpolarize**)
11. Descending regulation of pain: Some nociceptive ALS fibers synapse in midbrain(spinomesencephalic) and reticular formation of pons/medulla(spinoreticular) => descending **serotonergic**(from periaqueductal grey(**nucleus raphe magnus**)) and **noradrenergic** (**locus coeruleus**) VIA the **lateral** and **anterior funiculi of spinal cord** onto **opioidergic interneurons** in dorsal horn, which release **enkephalin.**
12. Neuroexams: Pain(sharp/dull), Temp(hot/cold)
13. HEADACHE – not from brain
14. Aspirin: ↓CycloOxygenase=>↓Prostaglandins=>↓sensitization.
15. ACUPUNCTURE - ↑release of opioid peptides, ↑hypothalamic/pituitary neurotransmitters/hormones, alter immune function
16. OPIOIDS: painkillers
17. SURGICAL pain management: in terminal cancer patients: **dorsal rhizotomy** (↓DRG).

22. Visual System

1. Optic Disk(papilla over lamina cribrosa), Fovea(↑#cones), Macula(visual acuity)
2. **Refractive power: 1/focus(m) (Diopters).** Cornea=42D, Lens($13D_{flat}$-$26D_{round}$) - modulation of refractive power (plasticity) in accommodation by ciliary muscle(PNS, constrict for closer image).
3. **Ciliary** muscles: PNS: from **Edinger-Westphal nucleus of CNIII – Ciliary ganglion – Short ciliary nerves->** Ciliary muscle
4. **Presbyopia** – inability to focus on close objects with age.
5. **Visual Acuity:** depends on **density** of photoreceptors and optical apparatus
6. **Pupil Diameter:** SNS(dilation) vs PNS(constriction)
7. Sympathetics: from Superior Cervical Ganglion- postganglionic follow Internal Carotid Artery-Opthalmic a.->Iris's **Dilator Pupillae Muscle.**
8. Parasympathetics: from Edinger-Westphal n. of CNIII->Ciliary ganglion->short ciliary nn->**Constrictor Pupillae muscle**
9. **Emmetropia** – normal sightedness, optical apparatus matches the length of the eyeball.
10. **Myopia** – nearsightedness, far images focus **in front** of retina (apparatus too strong or eyeball is too long). Use –D lens.
11. **Hyperopia** – farsightedness, far images focus **behind** the retina (apparatus too weak or eyeball is too short). Use +D lens
12. $20_{you}/20_{normal}$
13. **Papilledema** - ↑intracranial pressure=> ↓venous drainage=>dilation of retinal veins=> optic disk is pushed forward and white (not pink)
14. **Detached Retina** – from pigmental epithelium=>**scotoma,** can stop further by laser.
15. **Macular Degeneration** – neovascular, extreme myopia, some infections. Treat with **Photocoagulation – low%.**
16. **Diabetic Retinopathy** - ↑Glucose=>scotomas(severe if at macula), ↓permeability of basal membrane, aneurysms.

23. The Retina

1. Rods: synapse through **rod spherules,** sensitive to light(↑signal amplification), low resolution(highly convergent pathways)
2. Cones: synapse through **cone pedicles,** less sensitive to light(↓signal amplification), high resolution (less convergent pathways)
3. Rods/Cones release **Glutamate** at **NO light**(ie No stimulus). Recycle their outer pigmented disks (phagocytosed by **retinal pigment epithelium)**
4. RODS: Rhodopsin= Opsin(made, 7TM) + Retinal(derived from VitA(beta-carotene, **chromophore,** covalently attached to 7th TM segment))
5. **DARK current:** Rhodopsin(inactive) is coupled to **G protein**(inactive) =>↓**cGMP phosphodiesterase** =>↑cGMP=>cGMP-gated channels **open**=> depolarized membrane=> Glutamate released.
6. **Transducin** – cGMP binding protein involved in Phototransduction.
7. **Phototransduction:** light absorbed by visual pigment=>cis-retinal->all-trans-retinal=>↑cDMP phosphodiesterase=>↓cGMP (->↑5'GMP)=>closed cGMP-gated channel=> hyperpolarized=>↓glutamate release
8. **Visible** Electromagnetic spectrum: 400-700nm wavelength
9. 3 cones: $S_{hort\ wavelength}$/Blue/430nm, $M_{edium\ wavelength}$/green/530nm, $L_{ong\ wavelength}$/Red/560nm.
10. **NOTE:** all cone types are stimulated by all wavelength with **peaks** being specific.
11. **NOTE:** light reflected from natural objects is **not** monochromatic.
12. **5 retinal cell types: photoreceptors[Horizontal cells**-inhibitory, outer plexiform plexus] - **Bipolar cells** – [**Amacrine cells**-inner plexiform plexus]**Ganglion cell.**
13. Only Ganglion cell produce Action potentials(axons to **LGN**), others- graded potentials
14. **Bipolar Cells: OFF** type(Glutamate activates **ionotropic Receptor,** depolarize – sign conserving synapse), **ON type** (Glutamate inhibits **metabotropic Receptor,** hyperpolarize –sign converting synapse).
15. **Antagonistic Surround of Bipolar cells:** activated photoreceptors in **periphery of receptive field** form excitatory synapses on **Horizontal cells,** which inhibitory synapse on Bipolar(and others) cell in the **centre of receptive field** for that cell.
16. **Ganglion cells also have ON**(receive from ON Bipolar)/**OFF**(receive from OFF Bipolar) **types** and **Center Surround Organization of Receptive field.**
17. NOTE: Bipolar cells have only **excitatory** effect on Ganglion cells (ie ON excites ON..)
18. RETINITIS PIGMENTOSA: rods degenerate, ↓peripheral/night vision('tunnel'). Associated with ↓phagocytosis of shaded disks by retinal pigment epithelium
19. **Nyctalopia**(night blindness) - ↓VitA
20. **Color blindness** – common Red/Green blindness, X-linked Recessive: **Protanopia**(L cone/red absent), **Deuteranopia**(M cone/green absent). Low S cone –RARE
21. To test for colorblindness- use pseudo-isochromatic color plates.

24. Visual Pathways

1. Information from 4 visual quarters (Sup/Inf, Nasal/Temporal) follows different pathways to primary visual cortex.
2. Visual field is reversed on retina: L-R AND Sup-Inf.
3. Retinal Ganglion-> Optic nerve-> synapse in LGN(relay in thalamus to visual cortex), **Suprachiasmatic nucleus**(hypothalamus – circadian), **Pretectal nucleus**(midbrain, pupillary light reflex), **Superior Colliculus**(midbrain, eye movements).
4. Overlap between L/R visual fields=>**binocular vision,** + some peripheral regions do not overlap=>**monocular**
5. **Left Superior quadrant of Visual field:** LEFT eye: ->nasal-inferior retina->optic chiasm->Right LGN->Temporal optic radiation->Inferior portion of Primary Visual Cortex(V1) under the **calcarine sulcus**; RIGHT eye: temporal-inferior retina-NOT cross-> Right LGN->Temporal optic radiation->Inferior portion of Primary Visual Cortex(V1) under the **calcarine sulcus**
6. **Left Inferior quadrant of Visual field:** same as above upto Right LGN-> **Parietal** optic radiation->**Superior** portion of V1 above the **calcarine sulcus.**
7. **Right Half of Visual field:** same as above only Left->Right
8. **V1** –Broadman's 17, around occipital pole laterally, above and below calcarine sulcus medially
9. **V1-** blood supply from Posterior Cerebral (calcarine branch) + a bit from Middle Cerebral.
10. **Macular** region of Visual field is represented closer to **Occipital Pole** in V1
11. **Peripheral** region of visual field is represented closer to **Parieto-Occipital sulcus**
12. **Macular** retinotopic map>>Peripheral retinotopic map of V1.
13. Columnar Organization of V1 – Ocular Dominance Columns(contralateral and ipsilateral columns(6 layers from pia to arachnoid) alternate across cortex) + Orientation Columns(to horizontal/vertical direction of light, again across all 6 layers)
14. Parallel pathways originate from retinal ganglion cells: **Magnocellular neurons**(Depth/motion) from **M ganglion cell** synapse in 2/6 layers of LGN -> layer 4 of V1->**Dorsal(parietal) pathway.**
15. Parallel pathways originate from retinal ganglion cells: **Parvocellular neurons**(Shape/colour) from **P ganglion cells** synapse in other 4/6 layers of LGN -> layer 4 of V1-> **Ventral (inferior temporal) pathways.**
16. Neuroexam of visual field: 'Confrontation visual field test"
17. HEMIANOPIA: loss of one half of visual field
18. QUADRANTIC ANOPIA: loss of one quadrant of visual field
19. HOMONYMOUS anopia – same visual field loss in both eyes
20. HETERONYMOUS anopia – different defect in visual field loss for both eyes.(ex Bitemporal hemianopia)

25. Eye Movement

1. Movements: Conjugate(**Saccadic**('jump'), **Vestibulo-ocular**(head moves), **Optokinetic** reflex(smooth pursuit, head stationary, visual field moves) + Non-conjugate(di/con**Vergence**)
2. **SO4, LR6,** rest by III
3. **Nuclei:** in midbrain Tegmentum(III at level of Superior Colliculus; VI at level of Inferior colliculus) and Lower pons(IV close to pontomedullary junction)
4. **Vertical** eye movements control centres(midbrain): **rostral interstitial nucleus of the medial longitudinal fasciculus** and **Superior colliculus**(general)
5. **Horizontal/Saccadic** movements(pons): **pontine paramedian reticular formation**
6. **Optokinetic/smooth pursuit** movements (cerebellum): **vestibule-cerebellum**(flocculo-nodular lobe).
7. **+ nuclei** between pons and medulla also contribute to eye movements.
8. **Cortical Control Units: Frontal Eye field**(area8, planning/initiation of saccadic eye movements) + **Parieto-Occipital eye field**(area 7b/19, receives **dorsal pathway** from V1 about motion and depth info=> output related to optokinetic movements)
9. **Saccadic eye movements:** 900°/sec, no visual feedback.
10. **Frontal eye field**->down to pons, cross the midline, synapse on **pontine paramedian reticular formation(PPRF)**->output synapse on **abducens nucleus**=>(common final pathway of all conjugate horizontal eye movements) **2 outputs:** to ipsilateral abducens nerve(lateral rectus) + cross&ascend in **medial longitudinal fasciculus(MLF)** to contralateral oculomotor(medial rectus) =>gaze to one side horizontally.
11. **Neuroexam: H test**
12. Trochlear nerve palsy: ↓SO=> Inferior Oblique unopposed in medial gaze.
13. Oculomotor palsy: eye is down and out, ptosis, mydriasis(pupil dilation)
14. **Diplopia**(double lesion)
15. **Subtle** deviation in focus: use **Red Glass** test: red filter on one eye, observe white light.
16. INTERNUCLEAR OPHTHALMOPLEGIA: lesion in MLF=> ipsilateral eye does not adduct in lateral gaze, BUT convergence is fine.
17. PPRF lesion: since before the abducens nucleus=>both eyes cannot towards the side of the lesion in lateral gaze.
18. **One-and-a-Half** Syndrome: PPRF and MLF on same side is down=> both eyes do not move in ipsilateral lateral gaze AND only one eye(contralateral) moves in contralateral lateral gaze.

26. Vestibular System

1. Endolymph(rich in K^+, low on Ca^{2+}) movement detected by the **Stereocilia** of the hair cell. Vesicles released at the base of the cell into the synapse with afferents of CN VIII.
2. Endolymph movement deflects stereocilia and cause **either** Depolarization **or** Hyperpolarization (graded potentials) of membrane (α on direction). Deflection towards longer stereocilia causes stretch of the **tip links** between stereocilia and Open **mechanically gated K+ channel** (remember endolymph is rich in K+) =>depolarization=>↑Ca influx=>vesicle release.
3. Linear Acceleration transduced by Otolith organs(Utricle, Saccule – calcium carbonate crystals on cilia, oriented in opposite direction around **striola**).
4. Angular Acceleration transduced by Semicircular canals (horizontal, Ant Vertical, Post Vertical – hair cells(crista) inserted into cupula (in Ampulla of semicircular canal) in endolymph)
5. **Utricle – kinocilium**(longest cilium?) is oriented <u>towards</u> the striola on either side of it.
6. **Saccule – kinocilium** is oriented <u>away</u> from striola on either side of it
7. **5&6=>** movement of otoliths would activate some fibers and inactivate others at the same time
8. Vestibular system operates at subcortical level, ie there is no primary vestibular cortex area.
9. Some vestibular projections reach Hypothalamus(nausea, sweating, ↑HR).
10. Most vestibular afferents: afferent limb of reflexes: Vestibulo-Ocular, Vestibulo-Spinal.
11. Afferents coming to Lateral Vestibular Nucleus project to Cerebellum and Limb Motor neuron
12. Afferents coming to Medial Vestibular Nucleus project in MLF to Extraocular Motor neurons and Back/Neck Motor neurons
13. Horizontal **Vestibulo-Ocular reflex**: Cupulas are on medial side of Horizontal canals with Kinocilium towards the back. Head rotation produce counter current of endolymph in the canals and either stretch/activate kinocilium (on ipsilateral side) or compress/deactivate it (on contralateral side).
14. Fibers from the **ACTIVATED** labyrinth enter brainstem at ponto-medullary junction and synapse in the **vestibular nucleus**->CROSS and synapse in **contralateral** abducens nucleus =>common final pathway for horizontal eye movement(↑ipsilateral to abducens nucleus Lateral Rectus and CROSS to contralateral MLF upto oculomotor nucleus=>contralateral medial rectus)
15. I.E.: Head rotation activate ipsilateral labyrinth organ and vestibular nucleus, which project to **contralateral** abducens nucleus.
16. VOR does not require visual input=> active in darkness.
17. VOR eye speed upto 300°/sec
18. **Nystagmus** – slow(reflex) and fast(reset, saccadic circuitry; direction of nystagmus))
19. **VOR nystagmus** – physiological, slow phase opposite to rotation.
20. **Neuroexam of brainstem function: Oculocephalic Maneuver (Dolls eyes)**(test if pathway from medulla to midbrain is intact) + **Caloric Testing of VOR**(cold/hot water)
21. MENIERE's disease: ↓endolymph circulation=> dilation of compartments, degeneration of hair cells=>vertigo, tinnitus, sensorineural hearing loss.
22. Motion Sickness(KINETOSIS): discrepancy between vestibular and visual inputs=>nausea
23. Alcohol intoxication: alcohol in endolymph=>vertigo

24. Antibiotics(STREPTOMYCIN): accumulate in endolymph and damage cells
25. Lesion on one side of VOR only causes **pathological** nystagmus(slow towards damaged, fast towards normal side)

27. Ocular Reflexes

1. **Optokinetic reflex**: focus on moving image
2. info of depth and motion is brought to **parieto occipital eye field**, output fibers descend to **Pontine Nuclei** (different from PPRF)- Cross midline to contralateral **Vestibulocerebellum**(flocculo-nodular lobe)-to Vestibular nucleus-[vestibular reflex pathways]
3. Optokinetic Nystagmus: psl.
4. **Pupillary Light Reflex:** to protect retinas from light intensity.
5. light in one eye – some retinal ganglion axons in optic nerve do not synapse in LGN but pass to **Pretectal nucleus**, axons from pretectal nucleus synapse **bilaterally** on **Edinger-Westphal** nucleus of CN III (accessory nucleus, PNS)- BOTH Oculomotor nerves-**Ciliary ganglion**-Short ciliary nerves to **Pupil Constrictor muscle**.
6. **Corneal Reflex:** nociceptors in cornea- pain fibers with V1 if trigeminal nerve to Pons, descend to medulla, synapse in spinal nucleus of CN V, from V axons activate BOTH facial (VII) nuclei in lower pons=> orbicularis oculi => Blink
7. Neuroexam: OKN tape, shows lesion to parieto-occipital eye field
8. Bell's palsy: ↓VII

28. Auditory System

1. frequency(pitch, 20-20000Hz), intensity(pressure amplitude, loudness, dB=20log(p/po)
2. anatomy of the ear…
3. Sound amplification in middle ear due to: i) size difference between tympanic membrane to oval window (20:1); ii) Lever ratios of malleus, incus, stapes.
4. Fluid compartments of Inner ear: Scala tympani [Basilar membrane+organ of Corti] Scala Media(**stria vascularis - ↑K+;** tectorial membrane) [Reissner's membrane] Scala Vestibuli.
5. Fluid in inner ear is **not** compressed in waves (unlike air in sound transduction)
6. **Place code** : High frequency sound activate cell on the basilar membrane close to Oval window; Low frequency sounds activate cell on the basilar membrane closer to helicotrema.
7. Signal is also amplified in the inner ear (iii) by the **outer hair cells,** which shorten in depolarization.
8. There No Central lesions that produce **unilateral hearing loss.**
9. Lesion to Inferior Colliculus disrupts ability to localize sound.
10. Primary Auditory Cortex **A1** – 41/42 on transverse temporal gyrus of Heschl on superior surface of temporal lobe.
11. **Tonotopic** organization of A1: low frequencies more **rostrally/laterally**, High frequencies more **caudally/medially.**
12. **Columnar** organization of A1: EE-ExcInhib alternate
13. **Low frequency localization:** detect **Coincidence detection** in **Medial Superior Olive**(MSO) which detects **interaural** TIME difference by the properties of EPSP summations.
14. **High frequency localization:** detect **Interaural Amplitude differences** in **Lateral Superior Olive:** input from one ear activates ipsilateral Superior Olive AND contralateral **Trapezoid nucleus,** which inhibit Superior Olive on its side.
15. Neuroexam: basic (snap fingers- LOW frequency sound), Weber's(fork in middle of skull), Rinne's() Tuning fork tests
16. **Weber's test:** in conductive hearing loss, the sound is perceived from the **side of the disease**; in sensorineural hearing loss, the sound is perceived by the healthy side.
17. **Rinne's test on each ear:** compare times for bone conduction(at mastoid) vs air conduction(amplified): normal:air>bone ; conductive loss: bone>air.
18. OTOSCLEROSIS: stapes fuses with oval window.=>conductive hearing loss
19. VESTIBULAR SCHWANNOMA: tumour compresses VIII in internal auditory meatus=>sensorineural hearing loss.
20. Lost hair cells (age, loud sounds) =>Sensorineural hearing loss =>Cochlear implants.

29. Chemical Senses

1. **Gustatory System:**
2. Taste receptors(**inotropic**[salt/sour]/**metabotropic**[sweet/bitter]) in taste buds of the tongue, no axons. Basal cells differentiate to receptors in the bud.
3. **Salt receptor:** Na enters **Amiloride-sensitive Na channel**=>depolarization=>↑Ca=>↑vesicle
4. **Sour receptor:** H+ either 1) enter **Amiloride-sensitive Na channel** or 2) Block K_{out} channel =>depolarization=>↑Ca=>↑vesicle release.
5. **Sweet receptor:** binds a sweet molecule=>↑AC=>↑cAMP=>close K channel=>depolarization=>↑Ca=>↑vesicle release
6. **Bitter receptor:** bind bitter molecule=> ↑PLC=>↑IP3/DAG=>↑Ca=>↑Na current in=>depolar.
   ALSO bitter molecule may block K channel=>depolarization
7. **Japanese: 5th taste: UMAMI from Monosodium Glutamate.**
8. **Gustatory pathway** (does NOT cross): **VII**(anterior 2/3, geniculate ganglion), **IX**(posterior 1/3, inferior ganglion of IX), **X**(posterior, inferior ganglion of X) afferents enter brainstem at ponto-medullary junction and synapse in **nucleus of solitary tract**, from there 2nd order fibers synapse in **Ventral Posterior Medial (VPM) nucleus of THALAMUS,** 3rd order fibers synapse in Primary Gustatory Cortex- Insular Lobe/lower part of postcentral gyrus.
9. **Olfactory system:**
10. Receptor cells in olfactory epithelium send axons (NOTE: no synapse like in gustatory) with **olfactory nerve** (CNI) covered with **ensheathing cells** (NEITHER Schwann nor Oligodendrocyte) to **Olfactory bulb.** Basal Cells replace olfactory epithelium every 60 days.
11. **Odour Receptor**(metabotropic): bind odorant to G-protein linked receptor, Gα(GTPase) activate AC=>↑cAMP=>open cation channels=>↑Na, Ca=>graded potential=>AP
12. **10000** odorants activate 1000 receptors, each in different way. **Same type** receptors project to same **glomerulus** of olfactory bulb.
13. There are **Horizontal inhibitory interneurons** between the glomeruli that allow 'subtraction' of signals.
14. Output cells (tufted/mitral) from the olfactory bulb send axons in **lateral olfactory tract** to directly (NOT through Thalamus) synapse in Olfactory cortex areas: **Piriform cortex, Peri-amygdaloid cortex, Entorhinal cortex** – all in Temporal lobe around Uncus.
15. Olfactory cortex has close relationship to Limbic system (emotions, amygdala)
16. **Vomeronasal Organ:** in Vomer bone: pheromone sensor. Bipolar neurons like in olfactory
17. HYPOGEUSIA: ↓taste: ↓salivary gland=>taste bud destruction
18. AGEUSIA: Loss of taste: 1)Bell's palsy at chorda tympani, 2)Wallenberg's syndrome – occlusion of PICA=> infarction of lateral medulla.
19. HYPOSMIA: ↓smell:=> affects taste
20. ANOSMIA: loss of smell: compression of olfactory tract by tumours
21. OLFACTORY HALLUCINATIONS: in partial epileptic seizures close to uncus.

Module E. Motor Systems.

30. Organization of the Motor System

1. Voluntary tracts **(4)**: Corticobulbar, Corticospinal, Rubrospinal, Reticulospinal
2. Involuntary tract **(2)**: Vestibulospinal tracts (receive sensory from vestibular nuclei only, **NOT** influenced by motor cortex, ALL other tracts receive info from cotex)
3. Start of <u>Motor Pathways</u>(7): **Lateral Corticospinal**(pyramidal layer 5 in precentral gyrus), **Corticobulbar**(pyramidal layer 5 in precentral gyrus), **Rubrospinal**(Red nucleus in midbrain), **Lateral vestibulospinal**(lateral vestibulospinal nucleus in Pons), **Medial vestibulospinal**(medial vestibulospinal nucleus in Pons/Medulla), **Pontine**$_{\text{medial reticulospinal}}$(Oral/caudal reticular nuclei in Pons), **Medullary**$_{\text{lateral reticulospinal}}$(Gigantocellular reticular nucleus in Medulla).
4. Motor tracts (6 long): **Ventromedial**(Pontine, Lateral vestibulospinal, Medial vestibulospinal), **Lateral**(Lateral corticospinal, Rubrospinal, Medullary reticulospinal) pathways.
5. Motor neuron distribution in **Ventral horn**: Dorsal(<u>flexor</u>/adductor, hence the 3 <u>Lateral</u> pathways), Ventral(extensor/abductor, hence the 3 <u>Ventromedial</u> pathways), Lateral(distal muscles-limbs), Medial(proximal muscle-trunk)
6. 2 of The three <u>Lateral</u> pathways innervate ipsilateral flexor motor neurons, but **Medullary reticulospinal tract** innervates motor neurons **bilaterally.**
7. LOWER motor neuron disease: **Amyotrophic Lateral Sclerosis**(Lou Gehrig's; ↓lower motor neurons, then pyramidal tract, then precentral gyrus destroyed=>muscle weakness, difficulty speaking/swallowing/breathing, No problem with sphincter control, sensory, intellect. Die within 3-5yrs of diagnosis from respiratory insufficiency/ aspiration pneumonia(↓cough reflex))
8. SPINAL cord disease: may affect cells and tracts of both motor and sensory pathways: **Anterior Spinal Artery Syndrome:** occlusion ↓ant 2/3 of cord=>↓2nd order motor neuron, Lateral/Anterior corticospinal tract, Anterolateral System(sensory) => paraplegia(↓LMN[anterior horn] or UMN[@pyramidal tracts]), risk of pulmonary emboli, infection(bladder/lung/decubitus ulcers). <u>Symptoms:</u> spastic paraparesis, bilateral Babinski, bilateral loss of pain/temp below lesion (other sensory OK), retention of urine, ↓sexual function.;;;
Central Medullary Syndrome: syringomyelia(cyst in central canal) usually in ventral part of cervical cord=>pressure on ventral horn and anterior commissure=> segmental muscle atrophy(hand/finger), pain/temp loss. <u>Symptoms:</u> stiffness in back/shoulders/arms/legs, headaches, ↓sweating, sex, bladder/bowel control.

31. Corticospinal & Corticobulbar fibers

1. **Corticospinal tract**: Prefrontal Cortex(planning)→PreMotor Cortex(area6,program)→ Primary Motor cortex(4,execution)→Lower motor neuron(direct or via interneurons)
2. **Homunculus** – somatotopic organization of primary cortex.
3. Premotor cortex projects to Motor cortex + directly to motor neurons; Medial portion is **Supplementary Motor Area.**
4. Both Premotor and Motor cortices receive input from **Posterior Parietal Area(5&7**, integrates sensory for motor planning), **Basal Ganglia**(via Thalamus), and **Cerebellum**(via Thalamus).
5. Primary Motor cortex also receives input from Primary Somatosensory Cortex(3,1,2)
6. **Simple** finger flexion(Motor Cortex and Sensory Cortex active), **Complex** finger movements(+Medial premotor area (supplementary motor area) active), **Mental** imagining of finger movements(ONLY Supplementary motor area is active)
7. **Sensory Stimuli** activate Motor Cortex via thalamus/S1.
8. **External Sensory Stimuli** activate Lateral Premotor Area via S1 and Posterior Parietal cortex.
9. **Lateral Corticospinal Tract** – predominantly for distal flexor muscles of the limbs-output modified by info from Basal ganglia/Cerebellum (via Thalamus) – reach/walk
10. **Route** of Corticospinal Tract: Corona Radiata-Internal Capsule(posterior limb, axons from medial part of motor cortex are more posteriorly)-Crus Cerebri-Basilar pons-decussation(90%)-Lateral Corticospinal tract[**Glutamate**]-[**AMPA**]α/γ motor neurons/excitatory interneuron in Ventral Horn.
11. **10%** of fibers that do not cross in decussation form the **Ventral Corticospinal Tract**, which does not extend past Thoracic level.
12. Corticomuscular tract – UMN(V layer) + LMN(Ventral Horn)
13. LMN lesions: ipsilateral paralysis/paresis, **loss of reflexes**, loss of tone=>atrophy/wasting, **fasciculations**(spontaneous twitches-characteristic of denervated muscle –fibrillations in EMG). EX: Amyotrophic Lateral Sclerosis, Peripheral nerve damage.
14. UMN lesions(above/below decussation): Initial Flaccid Paralysis(**spinal shock),** after a few weeks spinal function regained=>Spastic Paralysis, +Babinski, Hyperreflexia
15. BROWN-SEQUARD syndrome: hemisection of spinal cord: ipsilateral UMN lesion **below**(Spastic paralysis), ipsilateral LMN lesion **at** the site of hemisection(Flaccid/Areflexia), contralateral Pain/Temp loss (ALS), ipsilateral touch/vibr/proprioception (Dorsal Column-ML)
16. NOTE above that muscle analysis can reveal the level of hemisection.
17. **Paraplegia**: bilateral spinal cord injury from contusion/compression/laceration=>UMN↓ on both sides, ↑deep tendon reflex/clonus, urine retention/bladder distension(painless), ↓all sensory.
18. **Corticobulbar** fibers – to Cranial nerve Nuclei=>muscles of face and neck.
19. **Infarction of Posterior Limb** of Internal capsule=>↓Corticospinal, Corticobulbar, DC-ML, ALS=> for XII- contralateral tongue deviation; for Fibers that project to contralateral PPRF on lower pons=> ipsilateral eye deviation(due to one sided tonicity from other PPRF); for VII- contralateral **lower** facial paralysis (Upper VII nucleus receives input from BOTH sides, lower –only from contralateral); In peripheral VII damage – the whole side of the face is paralyzed!

32. Other Motor Pathways.

1. **Rubrospinal Tract** (flexors of proximal arms): Motor Cortex[Corticorubral tract] + fibers from cerebellar nuclei synapse on ipsilateral **Red Nucleus**(midbrain) -> CROSS in ventral portion of midbrain->Rubrospinal tract(lateral) to Cervical segments-α/γ motor neurons => voluntary flexion movement of the arms.
2. **Medullary$_{lateral}$ Reticulospinal Tract**(Distal Flexors): Each **Reticular nuclei** in medulla receives input from cortex bilaterally[**Corticoreticular fibers**] +sensory input from collateral ALS fibers of Spinoreticular tract(few fibers). From the reticular nucleus **some fibers cross/some don't** and travel in the spinal cord, synapsing on **interneurons,** which activate α/γ motor neurons of flexors=> facilitate limb flexor contractions.
3. **Pontine$_{medial}$ Reticulospinal Tract**(Proximal Extensors): Each **Reticular nuclei** in Pons receives input from cortex bilaterally[**Corticobulbar fibers**] +sensory input from collateral ALS fibers of Spinoreticular tract(most of the input). From the reticular nucleus fiber DO NOT CROSS and travel through medulla to spinal cord, synapsing on **interneurons,** which activate mainly γ motor neurons(some α) of extensors=> facilitate limb/trunk extensor contractions.
4. **Spinoreticular Tract**(Sensory): collateral fibers from ALS system excitatory synapse on medullary/pontine reticular nuclei and bring info about pain/temp/crude touch in the trunk/limbs.
5. **Lateral Vestibulospinal Tract**(Extensors): **Lateral Vestibular nucleus** in pons receives excitatory info from vestibular organs/ cerebellum +inhibitory info from cerebellar purkinje cells. From the vestibular nucleus fibers DO NOT CROSS and travel through medulla to spinal cord, synapsing on excitatory **interneurons**, which activate α motor neurons of trunk/limb extensors ('antigravity') =>keep balance
6. **Medial Vestibulospinal Tract**(Extensors): **Medial Vestibular nucleus** in pons receives excitatory info from vestibular organs/ cerebellum. From the vestibular nucleus fibers DO NOT CROSS and travel through medulla to spinal cord(cervical/upper thoracic level) in Medial Longitudinal Fasciculus with inhibitory(Glycine) synapse on α motor neurons of extensor muscles of back/neck=>stabilize head.
7. **'Gamma Loop'** – muscle spindles detect the positive change in muscle length. When muscle relaxes the spindle is stretched (slack) and can't determine further muscle changes, therefore γ motor neurons innervate contractile ends of the spindle to adjust to new length (mainly Medial Reticulospinal tract).
8. IN Myotatic reflex, **Ia** from muscle spindle activate α motor neuron of same muscle. (**Ib** from Golgi tendon organs)=> **!!!stimulation from Medial(pontine) Reticulospinal Tract will cause muscle contraction** by activating myotatic reflex arch.
9. DECORTICATE POSTURING: lesion above Red Nucleus=>↓Corticorubral, Corticospinal(↓flexion), Corticobulbar (↓Cranial nerves motor)=> flexed arms/extended lower limb(but flexed wrists/ plantar flexed feet) - (intact Rubrospinal/Medullary/Pontine Reticulospinal/Vestibulospinal tracts): in the arms Flexor input from Rubrospinal tract is stronger than extensor from Pontine Reticulospinal/Vestibulospinal tracts; in the leg there is no Rubrospinal tract=>extension.

10. DECEREBRATE POSTURING: lesion <u>below</u> Red Nucleus=> ~decorticate + ↓Rubrospinal=>no flexion of the arms=> extended arms/legs (but flexed wrists/ plantar flexed feet)

33. Muscle Innervation & Motor Unit.

1. Muscle Afferents: from **Muscle Spindle** (length/rate of change), **Golgi**(tension), thermo/nociceptors
2. **Muscle Spindle** – more in fine movement muscles. 2-12 intrafusal fibers. Contractile(myelinated motor supply-**Aγ**) + Non-contractile(myelinated sensory output, **Ia/II**) parts.
3. Intrafusal fibers: **Nuclear Bag** Fibers(nuclei in central bag; dynamic$_{length+RATE}$ + static$_{length}$) + **Nuclear Chain** Fibers(nuclei in a row; ~static).
4. Nuclear Dynamic bag is innervated by only Ia afferent, while Static and Nuclear chain by **Ia and II**.
5. Extrafusal fibers are innervated by large myelinated **Aα** fibers(fast conducting).
6. Stretch reflex – Ia from spindle excite homonymous Aα and through interneurons inhibit Aα of reciprocal muscle.
7. In sustained stretch muscle spindles are continuously excited.
8. α & γ activated simultaneously to prevent spindle 'unloading'.
9. **Golgi Tendon organ** – between tendon and extrafusal fibers (in series vs parallel muscle spindles). **Ib** sensory fibers ↑firing with ↑tension.
10. **Ib** through interneurons inhibit homonymous muscle/activate reciprocal Aα=> at contraction, fibers with large tension are OFF=>even distribution of tension among all fibers. Also at large tensions, **inverse myotatic reflex** is activated.
11. **Motor Control system:** Cortex, Brainstem, spinal cord + **Basal Ganglia/Cerebellum**
12. Aα motor neuron originates in spinal cord, has a collateral that innervates interneurons(**Renshaw cells**).
13. Motor neuron pools (~100 nuclei supplying the same muscle) are in columns spanning several cord segments in ventral horn.
14. **Motor Unit:** neuron -NMJ in centre of number of muscle fibers(α on fine movement): **TypeI**(slow-twitch, low tension, fatigue resistant, aerobic, small motor neuron/axon), **TypeIIA**(fast, large tension, fatigue-resistant, somewhat aerobic, large motor neuron/axon); **TypeIIB**(fast, large tension, rapidly fatigued, anaerobic, large neuron/axon)
15. **Force** of contraction α firing rate, number of units recruited.
16. HYPOTONIA: reduced tone: test with resistance to passive stretch (Ia or Aα, or other UMN problems)
17. LOWER MOTOR UNIT syndrome: damage to nuclei or axons: atrophy of muscle, ↓reflex/voluntary activation, fasciculations, fibrillations.

34. Diseases of the NMJ & Motor Unit.

1. Muscle weakness: Neurogenic or Myogenic(myopathic)
2. **Sites** of Lesion in Motor Unit: Soma (Lou Gehrig's disease[amyotrophic lateral sclerosis], Poliomyelitis), Axon (neuropathy, toxins, drugs, axotomy=>muscle replace with fibrous CoT), Schwann cells (Guillain-Barre syndrome, Diphtheria=>conduction slowing/block), Nerve ending (Botulism, Lambert-Eaton disease), Synaptic cleft (↓ACh Esterase), End plate (Myasthenia gravis, nACh-release defects), Muscle fiber (myotonias, muscular dystrophy).
3. Nerve ending: BOTULISM: toxin(protease) from anaerobic bacteria, *Clostridium botulinum*=>↓Ach exocytosis. Get Botulinum from food, infection, ingest spores from bacteria.
4. Nerve ending: Alpha-Latrotoxin: from black widow spider, causes massive release of Ach=>tetanus
5. Nerve ending: Beta-Bungarotoxin: ↓ACh exocytosis.
6. Nerve ending: Curare (delta-tubocurarine): nondepolarizing muscle relaxant, blocks AChR on postsynaptic membrane of NMJ.
7. Nerve ending: Lambert-Eaton syndrome: insufficient ACh release=>weakness improves with contin muscle contraction. α Oat cell carcinoma of lung (paraneoplastic syndrome). Signs/tests: reduced EPP (minEPP unchanged!), reflexes decreased. Treat with plasma exchange, Calcium Gluconate, 4-Aminopyridine.
8. Synaptic Cleft: **Congenital Myasthenia** (↓ACh-esterase=>↑EPP; Prolonged opening of AChR=>depolarization block=>muscle weakness, rapid fatigue, progressive atrophy; Abnormal ACh binding to R; Brief opening of AChR)
9. Synaptic Cleft: **Myasthenia Gravis:** autoimmune against ARChERs=>↓#AChR, Wider synaptic cleft, Smaller Junctional folds. Weakness improves with rest and worsens through muscular activity. αThymus tumor. => vision problems(double vision, ptosis), swallowing problems, EMG has a waning pattern, Tension test is positive(ACh-esterase inhibitor). Treat with Neostigmine/Pyridostigmine (ACh esterase inhibitor), Prednisone/Cortisone, Azathioprine/Cyclosporine(immunosuppressant), Plasma Exchange(temporary), Thymectomy. **Myasthenic crisis** –breathing difficulty, life threatening.
10. Synaptic cleft: **Myotonia congenita:** autosomal dominant disorder, Less Chloride channels expressed on muscle membrane=>slow relaxation of muscle=> increased excitability
11. **Myopathy: Muscular dystrophy: Duchenne:** ↓dystrophin in boys (X-linked)=>muscle weakness.
12. **LMN syndrome:** from viral infection, trauma, neurodegeneration.=>weakness/flaccid paralysis/↓tendon reflexes/atrophy, Fasciculations/Fibrillations(signs of denervation)
13. **Fasciculation:** irregular spontaneous contractions of muscle fibers in motor unit.
14. **Fibrillation:** spontaneous contraction of <u>single</u> muscle fibers.
15. **13,14**: in denervation AChR are spread over surface of the muscle (~fetus), and are sensitive due to voltage-gated Na/Ca channel=> twitches.
16. **Poliomyelitis:** infection with Poliovirus: direct contact, secretions(nose/mouth/feces)=>↓motor neurons of ventral horn. Prevent with immunization.

35. PNS disorders

1. **paresthesias** – abnormal sensation of burning, prickling, pin/needles, numbness
2. **ephapse** – parallel nerves contact and leak electrical impulses.
3. Signs of PNS lesion: -ve: weakness,↓tendon reflex, ANS deficit(sweat, ↓sensation; +ve: paresthesias due to ephaptic transmission, brief period of pain (trigeminal neuralgia) due to acute compression of the nerves - makes them hyperexcitable.
4. **Nerve Conduction Velocity**: Compression-slowing in CV of both motor/sensory, Demyelination - ↓↓CV of both motor&sensory, Mild axonal degeneration – slight ↓CV. Lesions to soma, NMJ, muscle do not produce change in CV.
5. **Damage** to peripheral nerve is from inside (axon) to outside (endo>peri>epineurium).
6. **Carpal tunnel syndrome** – compression of median nerve due to irritation of tendons (women>men)
7. **Axotomy: Wallerian Degeneration** of distal part, **Anterograde/Retrograde Transneuronal** degeneration – nerves distal/proximal to the damaged nerve.
8. **Regeneration(PNS)**: axonal sprouting from proximal part of damage under signals (nerve growth factor, laminins, adhesion molecule) from Schwann cells find the 'tube' built by Schwann and reconnect
9. **Regeneration(CNS)**: rare: oligodendrocytes do not release NGF, nor form guiding tubes; Astrocytes multiply at lesion and form a glial scar **(Gliosis),** which blocks sprouting;+there are Inhibitory chemicals
10. **Reinnervation of denervated** skeletal muscle: regenerating axons differentiate into nerve terminals at the original synaptic sites: synaptic basal lamina has **Laminin11**, extrasynaptic BL has **Laminin2**.
11. Peripheral Neuropathy: **Guillain Barre Syndrome** (aka acute idiopathic polyneuritis, infectious polyneuritis, acute inflammatory polyneuropathy): following Respiratory/GI infection or autoimmune nerve inflammation leads to demyelination=>weakness. Test with NCV. EMG, CSF(for ↑protein). Treat with artificial ventilation, **Plasmapheresis**(plasma exchange), IV immune globulin to prevent respiratory failure, aspiration, pneumonia.
12. Peripheral Neuropathy: **Leprosy(Hansen's Disease)**:caused by *Mycobacterium Leprae*, most common treatable worldwide infection of skin and peripheral nerve. Treat with antibiotics.
13. Peripheral Neuropathy: **Diabetes Mellitus:** hyperglycemia causes polyneuropathy: sensory(symmetric start from legs), motor(asymmetric), autonomic
14. Peripheral Neuropathy: **Alcoholic Polyneuropathy:** due toxic effect or nutritional deficiency(thiamin). Symptoms are numbness, tingling, burning feet, weakness. Starts with sensory neuropathy from distal foot-leg..than motor losses. NCV is normal.
15. Peripheral Neuropathy: **Lead Poisoning:** NO sensory symptoms, bilateral weakness in arms/fingers(!); motor neuropathy in adults, encephalopathy in children.

36. Spinal Reflexes

1. **clonus** – rhythmic oscillations between flexion/extension
2. Monosynaptic reflex (deep tendon reflex/myotatic reflex), Polysynaptic reflex(one+ interneurons)
3. Stretch reflexes: Deep tendon, Golgi tendon(reverse myotatic), Flexion crossed extension
4. **Landmarks** for reflex testing: Inspiration(diaphragm-C3,4,5), Shoulder Abd(deltoid-C5), Elbow flexion(biceps-C5,6), Wrist extension(extensor carpi/radialies$_{long/brev}$-C6,7), elbow Extension(triceps, C7,8), Finger flexion(flexor digitorum$_{superficialis/profundus}$, C8), Finger Abd/Add(Interossei, C8,T1), Thigh add(Adductor$_{long/brevis}$, L2,3), Knee extension(Quads, L3,4), Great toe extension(Extensor hallucis longus, L5,S1), Ankle plantar flexion(calfs, S1,2), Anal contraction(sphincter ani externus, S2,3,4)
5. **Scale for reflex: 0-4**(Very brisk)
6. Stretch reflex: to maintain the muscle at a desired length determined by the descending pathways(corticospinal/corticobulbar). Muscles are always a bit stretched=>reflex maintains the muscle tone.
7. Inverse stretch reflex(aka Clasp-Knife reflex)- bisynaptic, slower than stretch reflex, function in protection of the muscle/tendon and Posture maintenance at the Quads level.
8. **Flexion Crossed Extension reflex:** pain fibers (Adelta/C) through a bunch of interneurons activate flexion of ipsilateral limb, extension of contralateral limb (ex: stepping on nail)
9. **Plantar response-Babinski**: normally in Adults flexion of toes, in children/lesion-extension/fanning
10. **UMN lesion**=>Hyperreflexia/Clonus, if lesion in spinal of cord, initially Areflexia, due to spinal shock
11. **Hyporeflexia**: LMN lesion, Spinal cord damage, ↓NMJ, Muscle lesion, Sensory loss, Peripheral nerve lesion

NEUROSCIENCE: The Most Rapid Review Of All Topics

Module F. Movement Disorders

37. Movement Disorders: Intro

1. **dyskinesia** – fragmentary/incomplete movement
2. **dysmetria** – improper measuring of distance in muscular acts
3. **dysdiadochokinesia** – inability to perform rapid alternating movements
4. **ataxia** – lack of finely tuned muscular movements for posture(lesion in cerebellum)
5. Movement disorders are hypo-(Parkinson) or hyperkinetic(Huntington), due impaired postural reflexes or impairment during movement. Disorders exhibit themselves as excessive involuntary movements, uncoordinated movements under voluntary control, or hypokinetic state where initiation is poor.
6. Involuntary movements: **Tremor**(normal 8-12Hz, Parkinson 5Hz), **Chorea**(irregular movements), **Athetosis**(slow writhing abnormal movement of limb/trunk/head)
7. Hypokinetic disorders result from lesions at NMJ, LMN, ↓basal ganglia(Parkinson's)
8. **Posture, Stance, Gait** reveal Disorders, since many systems are involved: **sensory**: visual/vestibular/proprioceptive; **motor**: cortex, supplementary motor cortex, basal ganglia, cerebellum,LMNs
9. Decorticate(lesion above red nucleus) vs Decerebrate(lesion at level of midbrain/pons
10. **Tremor: resting**(Parkinson), **essential**(postural, due to basal ganglia disorder, NOT Parkinsonian), **intention**(kinetic, due to cerebellar disorder)
11. **Akinesia in Parkinson's:** also see stooped posture; rigid, slow shuffling gait with poor swinging of the arms.
12. **Rigidity in Parkinson's:** 2 types of muscle stiffness: **'cogwheeling'**(ratcheting passive movement), **'leadpipe'**(continuous resistance to movement)
13. **Loss of postural reflexes in Parkinson's:** associated with difficulties in starting movements.
14. **Glabellar reflex:** repetitive tap on forehead should illicit blinking that normally stops after a while, but does NOT in Parkinson patients
15. **Parkinson stages:** 1.Unilateral, 2.Bilateral but with postural reflexes, 3.Bilateral with loss of postural reflexes, 4.Severe disability but some movement, 5.Akinesia
16. **Speech** is affected in Parkinson's disease
17. **HUNTINGTON's :** characterized by Chorea, Autosomal Dominant
18. Drug-induced Movement Disorders: **Tardive Dyskinesia**(antipsychotic drugs, movement of jaw, lips, tongue. Older people higher risk for permanent), **Dopa-induced dyskinesia**(side effect of L-Dopa in Parkinson patients, Choreic movements or dystonias(face grimace, eye closure))
19. Drug-induced Parkinsonism: drugs that block Dopamine receptors or deplete Dopamine stores. Relieved after stoppage of drug use.
20. **Dystonia**: partial or segmental muscle spasms or sustained postures:ex **Spasmodic torticollis**-dystonia of the neck, SCM hypertrophied
21. **Ballismus:** rapid, exaggerated, flinging, abnormal rotations of the limb.
22. **Hemiplegia**(accompanied by athetosis) →hemiplegic gait: one arm in flexed, ipsilateral leg extended.
23. **Tic Syndrome:** transient, coordinated movements: ex Eye blinking, arm jerks, head shaking, **Tourette's**(autosomal dominant, may show ADHD)

38. Movement Disorders: Basal Ganglia

1. Basal ganglia: αprefrontal, premotor, primary motor cortex, BUT no direct synapses with Motor neurons =>initiation/control of voluntary movement
2. Basal ganglia= Striatum(Caudate nucleus+putamen)+ Globus pallidus(external+internal) + Subthalamic nucleus(STN) +Substantia nigra(pars reticulata$_{[GABAergic]}$+pars compacta$_{[DOPA]}$)
3. Main output from BG is **inhibitory** drive on thalamus and cortex
4. **Motor loop: Cortex**[Glutamate'+']**Striatum**$_{medium\ spiny\ neurons}$[GABA'-']**GPi/SNr**[GABA'-']**Ventra- Lateral nucleus of Thalamus**['+']**supplementary motor area**(6)
5. SNr also GABA-inhibits VLnT (ie GPi+SNr – same function–tonically inhibit Thalamus=>↓Motor out);
6. **GPe** relays GABA-inhibition to **STN**
7. **STN** inreturn is glutamatergic onto GPi/SNr
8. **SNc is Dopaminergic**, with the metabolic byproduct, **Neuromelanin** accumulates with age in SNc cells – at autopsy can observe degeneration of SNc by loss of dark pigment.
9. **Medium spiny nerves in Striatum** have Dopamine receptors: inhibitory D2-R, and activating D1-R. Total Dopaminergic input reduces the phasically the inhibition from BG to Thalamic neurons!(thus if loose, inhibition increases)
10. **Extrapyramidal system**(circuits of BG) influence **Pyramidal System**(corticobulbar/corticospinal)
11. so, Striatal neurons have a **Direct Path** to GPi/SNr, which has D1 receptors for dopamine from **SNc** that excites the Direct pathway=>more inhibition on Thalamus=>less stimulation of Supplementary area 6=>**Facilitate movement**
12. also, Striatal neurons have an **Indirect Path,** which normally **Inhibits movement,** but has D2-Receptors for dopamine from SNc, which inhibits Striatum['-']GPe['-']STN['+']GPi/SNr path (indirect)=>↓inhibition of thalamus=> facilitate movement
13. **so**, motor signal from SMA(6) is shared between BG and Motor cortex, with BG(direct/indirect pathways +SNc) modulating the output via Thalamus.
14. **Thus, Degeneration** of any component above will cause disease: ex. ↓SNc=>↓Dopamine=>↓Direct path, ↑Indirect path=>↑GPi/SNr inhibition on Thalamus=>Akinesia, Bradykinesia, Muscular rigidity, Resting tremor of **Parkinson's patients** (hypokinetic), **bilateral**
15. ↓**Striatal neurons with D2-R's**=>↓inhibition of GPe in indirect path=>↑inhibition on STN=>↓activation of GPi/SNr=>↓inhibition on Thalamus=>↑↑movements, Chorea in **Huntington's** disease, bilateral involuntary movements of head,arms, legs, ↓mental state.
16. ↓**STN** (from stroke on one side)=>↓activation of GPi/SNr=> ↓inhibition of Thalamus=>**Hemiballismus** of contralateral side.
17. **Parkinsonism** – conditions that mimic Parkinson's disease, ie affect Dopamine pathways, while SNc is normal: i)**Drug-induced:** D2 blockers(PHENOTHIAZINES) for psychosis, RESERPINE(deplete dopamine stores), drugs with MPTP(damage SNc mitochondria), ii)**Vascular**: strokes affecting BG, iii)**Repetitive Head Trauma**: boxing dementia, iv)**Postencephalitic Parkinsonism**: viral induced SNc degeneration.
18. '**Huntingtonism**': other Choreas:i)**Sydenham's Chorea**: autoimmune inflammation of BG in 5-15yrs, easy to treat, ii)**Drug-induced:** L-DOPA, Anticonvulsants, Antipsychotic=>↑Dopamine activity
19. Parkinson(0.15%@55yrs) therapies: L-Dopa/Carbidopa(oral Sinemet)-Carbidopa inhibits Dopamine formation in Periphery, but NOT cross BBB, but with time ineffective, due to degeneration of SNc cells completely; Use

BROMOCRIPTINE(↑D2R) or PERGOLIDE(↑D1/D2-Rs), AMANTADINE(↑D release, but psychotic side effects), SELEGILINE(deprenyl, **MAO** inhibitor in early PD), ENTACAPONE/TOLCAPONE(**COMT** inhibitors=>↑D), BENZTROPINE(Muscarinic Antagonist, that inhibits Excitatory cholinergic interneurons that activate Striatum, helps with Tremor, NOT rigidity/hypokinesia, Side effects: confusion, Drowsiness,↑dementia), **Surgical** lesion of STN,GPi,Thalamus, Deep Brain stimulation (100Hz+)↑GABA on GPi

20. Huntington(0.01%@40yrs) **therapies**: none, use symptomatic treatment: antidepressants, HALOPERIDOL(D2R antagonist=>↓Choreic Movements, BUT ↓swallowing,speech,gait

39. Movement Disorders: Cerebellum

1. Cerebellum and Basal ganglia are Subcortical motor systems for coordination and learning of moves with NO direct innervation of Motor neurons.
2. Cerebellum ensures smooth movement by **Comparison** of descending/ascending signals, modifying **Timing** of descending signals, **Memory storage** of learnt moves via **Synaptic plasticity**.
3. 3 regions: **Cerebro-cerebellum**(lateral cerebellum receives from **deep pontine nuclei** for planning/monitoring moves), **Spino-cerebellum**(vermis/paravermis receives from spinal cord for body/limb move regulation), **Vestibulo-cerebellum**(flocculonodular lobe receives from Vestibular apparatus for balance/eye movements)
4. Cerebellar **peduncles: Superior**(cerebellum→midbrain/pons), **Middle**(pons→Cerebellum), **Inferior**(spinal cord/medulla→cerebellum, vestibular apparatus/lateral vestib nuclei ⇔ cerebellum,)
5. Cerebellar **cortex** 3 layers: Granule, Purkinje, Molecular cell layers with 2 fiber inputs: **Climbing** fibers from Inferior Olivary nucleus, **Mossy** from all other inputs; The only **output** from cerebellar cortex – **GABAergic Purkinje cells**, synapse in **Deep Cerebellar nuclei**(dentate, interpositus), which are excitatory on motor systems.
6. Motor loop: Motor cortex, Cerebellum, Thalamus. Halves of Cerebellum receive ipsilateral afferents and affect contralateral motor-**cortex** (ie ipsilateral motor function due to decussations=>**Ipsilateral Ataxia**)
7. Cerebro-Cerebellar Pathway: **SMA(6)**[via Pontine relay n/Inf Olivary n, Middle peduncle, CROSS, Glutamate'+']**Lateral Cerebellar cortex→Purkinje cells**[Inhibitory]**Dentate nucleus**[Superior peduncle, CROSS, Excitatory]**VLnT**[excite]**Motor Cortex(4)** see diagram on p 47-7
8. Spino-Cerebellar pathway: **4 ascending tracts**[inferior peduncle]**Vermis/paravermis cortex**['-'] **Interpositus nucleus**[Superior Peduncle, CROSS'+']**VLnT[+]M1**
9. Vestibulo-Cerebellar pathway: VIII[Inf Peduncle]Flocculo-Nodular lobe➔i) Bilateral **Medial Vestibular nuclei** via Superior Peduncle, which coordinate Head/eye movements via MVST(medial vestibulospinal tract), ii) ipsilateral **Lateral Vestibular nucleus** via Inferior Peduncle, which coordinates extensor limb movements(anti-gravity) via LVST
10. Cerebellar **lesions** cause: ipsilateral Ataxic Stance(feet wide stance), Ataxic Gait, Disorder of Posture/balance, **Dysarthria**(slurred/slow/monotonous speech), ↓Muscle tone(**Rebound phenomenon, poor myotatic reflex**), Limb ataxia(**Dyssynergia=dysmetria+dysdiadochokinesia**), Intention tremor, **Titubation**(head tremor, 3Hz), Nystagmus.
11. Lesion are due to Tumors(midline), Strokes(lateral), Toxins
12. **Cerebellar Tumor:** common in children, Astrocytoma=>↑ICP=>headache,vomit,papilledema, hydrocephalus; Wide-based stance, truncal ataxia, hypotonia, no balance, nystagmus
13. **Cerebellar Stroke:** one-sided=>ipsilateral limb, truncal ataxia, dysarthria, intention tremor, dyssynergia, rebound phenomenon, +brainstem signs: facial weakness, sensory loss
14. **Louis-Barr syndrome** (ataxia telangiectasia, gene11, AutoRecessive): loss of Purkinje cells in cerebellar cortex=>delayed motor/growth/sexual development, ↓humoral/cell-mediated immunity; see Ataxia, dysarthria, facial weakness, oculomotor↓; Death in 30yr
15. **Alcohol damage Anterior lobe of Cerebellum:** vermis+anterior↓ due to malnutrition=>loss of purkinje neuron, gliosis=>dysmetria in legs, truncal ataxia,

lurching gait, intention tremor of lower body, BUT NO Nystagmus, Dysarthria, Hypotonia.
16. **Anatomy- Disorder:** Vestibulo-cerebellum organizes head/eye moves to balance changes=>lesions cause imbalance, inability to walk heel-to-toe, nystagmus, Titubation, Head tilt;
17. Spino-cerebellum organizes posture/limb movement=> lesions cause imbalance, gait/arm ataxia;
18. Cerebro-cerebellum plans/times/learns movements=>lesions cause ataxia, intention tremor, ipsilateral hypotonia, decomposition of movements, ipsilateral dysdiadochokinesia/rebound phenomenon/dysmetria, dysarthria

Module G. ANS

40. Autonomic Nervous System

1. Hypothalamus(comparator) maintains Homeostasis by receiving **Neuronal**(CN's via Solitary nucleus) or Humeral(circumventricular organs) inputs.
2. ANS=PNS+SNS+ EntericNS
3. Enteric:Myenteric$_{Auerbach}$(gut motility)+Submucous$_{Meissner's}$(secretions) plexuses, modulated by SNS/PNS
4. SNS: preganglionic[ACh on nAChR]postganglionic[NE on AR]smooth muscle, glands, Cardiac muscle
5. PNS: preganglionic[ACh on nAChR]postganglionic[ACh on muscarinicAChR]smooth, cardiac, gland
6. SNS preganglionics synapse in Chain ganglia, Prevertebral ganglia(celiac, Sup mesenteric, Inf Mesenteric, Aorticorenal), Adrenal gland.
7. PNS preganglionics synapse in Ciliary, Pterygopalatine, Submandibular, Otic ganglia in head, and Terminal Ganglia in body organs.
8. Table p 48.14 – Adrenergic receptor types
9. ATENOLOL – Beta1 Antagonist used in Hypertension
10. SALBUTAMOL – Beta2 agonist used in Asthma (bronchodilator)
11. ATROPINE – muscarinic antagonist causes mydriasis
12. Hirschsprung's Disease (Megacolon) – absence of parasympathetic ganglia in distal colon.
13. Complex Regional Pain Syndrome (CRPS) – chronic pain after tissue injury(bone,soft,nervous) even after healing: Sympathetic hyperactivity, Sensitization of nociceptors to NE.

41. Hypothalamus

1. Hypothalamus controls 5 processes(BP/Electrolytes, Body T°C, Energy metabolism, Reproduction, Emergency response) via 3 integrative outputs (Autonomic, Endocrine, Motivation/Behaviour)
2. pheromones, Autocrine, paracrine, endocrine, neuroendocrine signalling
3. Hypothalamus zones: Periventricular (3rd ventricle), Medial(most nuclei), Lateral(most tracts)
4. **Anterior pituitary**(adenohypophysis from Rathke's pouch): Parvocellular neuroendocrine cells (paraventricular/arcuate nuclei) terminate on 1° Capillary plexus→portal vein→2° Capillary plexus in Ant Pituitary(**Tubero-Infundibular tract)**. Neurohormones that either ↑release of hormone(TRH, **CRH**, GnRH, GHRH), or inhibit it(Somatostatin(GH inhibiting), Prolactin inhibiting hormone).
5. In response AP releases GH, TSH, **ACTH**, FSH/LH, Prolactin, which may act on (3) glands: Thyroid gland, **Adrenal Cortex**(GFR,..**Cortisol**..), Gonads.
6. **Posterior pituitary**(neurohypophysis): Magnocellular neuroendocrine cells (paraventricular/supraoptic nucleus) terminate in posterior pituitary on fenestrated capillaries from **Inferior Hypophyseal Artery** (Supraoptico-Hypophyseal tract), releasing ADH(vasoconstriction/water resorption) or Oxytocin.
7. Regulation of **Feeding: Ventromedial nucleus**(↓feeding), **Lateral Hypothalamus**(↑feeding). Short term regulation is by Glucose levels, long term by **Leptin** on R's of **Arcuate nucleus,** which has inhibitory links to Lateral Hypothalamus
8. Regulation of **Water balance:** input from osmotic stimuli, vagus, mechano-sensitive receptors in vessels, Angiotensin at **Subfornical organ** cause ADH release and Motivational system→drinking
9. Regulation of **Temperature: Anterior Hypothalamus**(↓Temp, Has Temperature sensitive cells), **Posterior Hypothalamus**(↑Temp). Sensory input integrated and output to ANS for vasoconstriction/dilation, Motivation for seeking colder/warmer places
10. **Frohlich syndrome:** damage to Ventromedial Nucleus=> ↑feeding, obesity
11. **Diabetes Insipidus:** absence of ADH(lesion in supraoptic/paraventricular nuclei), interruption of supraopticohypophyseal tract=>excessive thirst/drinking, ↑urine
12. **Hypothermia:** lesion to Posterior Hypothalamus=>ant active=>↓metabolism, motor activity, peripheral vasodilation.
13. **Hyperthermia:** lesion to Anterior Hypothalamus

42. Autonomic Control Circuits

1. Autonomic control of **Pupil**: Hypothalamo-spinal fibers synapse on sympathetic cells in **intermediolateral** column, which activates papillary dilation.
2. Autonomic control of **Urinary Bladder**: under Sympathetic/Parasympathetic(internal sphincter/detrusor muscles) and Somatic Innervation(External Sphincter) with signals originating in Frontal cortex, Hypothalamus, and Pontine micturition centre(below tentorium cerebelli).
3. Filling of bladder: pressure receptors in the wall sent afferents, which synapse on Parasympathetic preganglionic fibers in the spinal cord, innervating bladder muscles; afferents also travel to pons/cortex.
4. Autonomic control of **Reproductive Organs:** input to cortex from sensory(olfactory, visual, sensory) and to spinal cord from genitalia and descending from brain. In spinal cord inputs innervate SNS/PNS directly/via interneurons or ascend to the brain. 'Point and Shoot'
5. **Circadian Rhythm:** daily pattern of activity(feeding) and inactivity(sleeping) modulating many PSL parameters via the internal biological clock, which without any Zeitgebers has 25 hour cycle. The clock is located in the **Suprachiasmatic nucleus** and receives resetting info from the photoreceptors in retina via the **retino-hypothalamic tract**; the output is **neuronal**(↑Melatonin from Pineal in dark) **and Humoral**(ADH from SCN)
6. **Horner's Syndrome:** miosis, ptosis, anhidrosis due ↓SNS at central lesion(transection of cervical cord), preganglionic lesion(lung tumor), or postganglionic lesion (@Internal Carotid, tumour in cavernous sinus)
7. **Automatic bladder:** transection of spinal cord->no voluntary control of bladder, only reflex
8. **Atonic Bladder:** lesion to dorsal nerve roots of sacral segments=>no sensation of fullness=>incontinence.
9. **Jet Lag:** west flight is easier to fix. Melatonin used 1hr before sleep.
10. **Sleep wake disorders in Blind:** no zeitgebers to reset internal clock
11. **Seasonal Affective Disorder (SAD):** decrease in day length, ↑melatonin in blood.

Module H. Selected topics

43. Sexual Differentiation of the Brain

1. Male/Female brain is different:i) Disease susceptibility, ii)Problem solving, iii)Hormonal environment(cyclic LH/FSH for females).
2. Most of Sexual Dimorphism is in Hypothalamus (Sexually Dimorphic Nucleus$_{M>F}$(**SDN**/INAH-**1**), Interstitial nuclei of the Anterior Hypothalamus(**INAH2,3,4**), Suprachiasmatic nucleus, Supraoptic nucleus, Paraventricular nucleus, Ventromedial nucleus) with some dimorphism also in Corpus callosum, Anterior Commissure.
3. The differences are morphological(size/number of neurons), in patterns of dendritic ramification, ratio of spiny synapses to non-spiny, transmitter content, uptake/release/synthesis, #enzymes, mRNA levels.
4. Not only male/female differences, but also Homosexual/Heterosexual ones exist: **INAH3 is smaller** in Women/Homosexual men, **SCN is larger** in Homosexuals than heterosexuals.
5. **Sexual differentiation**: genetic sex(Testes determining factor in Sex region of Y chromosome=>testes)=>gonad differentiation=> sex hormones cause body/brain differentiation.
6. Males-↑Testosterone, Females-↑estrogen, BUT only Testosterone is important in sex differentiation of body/brain via the appropriate receptor (↓ in **Androgen Insensitivity syndrome**)
7. Critical period in differentiation: 12-20weeks, in males there is ↑in testosterone, in females no peaks in any hormones.
8. Inside the cell Testosterone is converted to estradiol by Aromatase, which binds cytoplasmic receptor and acts as a transcription factor –ie indirect effect on neuronal signalling. There is also a direct effect that modulates NT release.
9. Hypothalamus contains ↑numbers of Estradiol Receptors.
10. Controversial: female fetus exposure to **Diethylstilbestrol** (synthetic estrogen to ↓spontaneous abortion) caused ↑SDN in females(usually ↑SDN in Males)=>↑%homosexuality in females.

44. Emotions

1. Hippocrates: blood(Sanguinic)+Mucous(Phlegmatic)+Yellow bile(Choleric)+Black bile(Melancholic)
2. Brain effect on emotions: **James-Lange theory**(smile=>happy), VS **Cannon-Bard Theory**(happy=>smile). Can fake facial expression, but can't fake emotions.
3. Broca's Limbic Lobe= Subcallosal gyrus+Cingulate gyrus+Isthmus+Parahippocampal gyrus+Uncus
4. **Papez Circuit of Emotions:** Hippocampal formation[Fornix]Hypothalamus[Mammilo-thalamic tract]Anterior Thalamic nuclei=>Cingulate Gyrus=>back to Hippocampal formation..
5. **Limbic system** expanded after MacLean on Papez'a frame: add amygdala, and there are projections to neocortex (p52-7).
6. **Case of Phineas Gage:** damage to **Frontal lobe**=>changed to erratic/undependable.
7. **Frontal Lobotomy:** in schizophrenics, but worse results after.
8. **Kluver-Bucy Syndrome:** removal of lateral lobes+amygdale=>tame, emotionless, ↑sexuality.
9. **Removal of Amygdala** causes reduction in fear (fear conditioning experiments on dogs, similar experiments with humans+imaging+ pictures of emotions)
10. **Neural Circuit of fear:** Input to Amygdala from Auditory Cortex AND <u>directly</u> from sensory neurons at **Basolateral nuclei;** output to Hypothalamus(ANS response), Periaqueductal grey matter(behaviour), and Cerebral cortex(Emotions).
11. **Anxiety Disorders:** panic, obsessive-compulsive, post-traumatic stress, **phobia** – due to Imbalanced input to Hypothalamus from Amygdala(↑input=>anxiety) and Hippocampus(↓input=>anxiety); also Frontal lobe is involved (Benzodiazepine(~GABA) sites↓ in Frontal lobe in panic disorders).
12. **Tumor** amygdale=>hostility/aggressive behaviour; Tumor in Hypothalamus=>fits of anger/deep sad.
13. **Psychomotor Epilepsy:** originate in temporal lobe: 1st get Olfactory/Gustatory hallucinations, then mood change(anxiety,loneliness)→dreamy state→motor phase(coordinated series of complex behaviours). When recovered, no recollection of what happened (memory down)

45. Consciousness

1. –ability to be aware of oneself and environment, and to respond appropriately to environmental stimuli
2. –depends on Synchronization of Cortical neurons, firing at 40Hz
3. Consciousness results from memory, learning, distinguishing self, **re-entry**(recursive comparison of info by different brain regions located in circuits of **thalamocortical** system.
4. Coma – non-sleep loss of consciousness for an extended period/deep state of consciousness
5. Levels of Consciousness: Lethargic, Obtunded, Stuporous, Comatose.
6. **Brainstem and Consciousness:** reticular formation in midbrain receives **collateral** connections from ascending pathways(spinothalamic tract, spinal tract of V, solitary tract, vestibular/cochlear nuclei, olfactory/optic system) and project via 2 branches: 1) to thalamus, modulating thalamic **relay** and **Intralaminar** nuclei, 2)nd branch penetrates Lateral hypothalamic area and joined by ascending output from Hypothalamic and Forebrain cells.
7. **Lesions** in either of 2 branches, thalamus, midbrain, or both cerebral hemisphere impair consciousness.
8. Brainstem plays a role for i)condition of consciousness, ii)Attentive vigilance, iii)Wake-sleep rhythm
9. ECG on Thalamic relay neurons: 2 states: **Transmission** mode(high Frequency(12+Hz)desynchronized pattern in wakefulness, resting potential is near Firing threshold, there is ACh-ergic input from rostral pons/basal forebrain) and **Burst** mode (low freq(3-Hz), synchronized pattern of hyperpolarized neurons in sleep/coma).
10. Vegetative state follows coma sometimes – lost ability to think/unaware of environment, but show normal sleep patterns and can perform non-cognitive functions.
11. Brain death: no ECG, no breathing/movement/reflexes: due to **Anoxia, Ischemia, Intracranial Hemorrhage, Trauma, Tumors, ↑ICP/uncal herniation.**
12. Locked-in-Syndrome: blockage of Basilar artery=>infarction of Pons=>complete paralysis of voluntary of all voluntary muscles except for Vertical eye movement.
13. Coma causes: Supratentorial mass lesions, Subtentoral lesions, Metabolic/Diffuse cerebral disorders
14. Glasgow Coma scale: 3-15. 8 is critical for coma: Best Eye4/Verbal5/Motor6 responses
15. Respiration is regulated by several centers of cortex and brainstem=>specific patterns with lesions: **Cheyne-Stokes respiration**(lesion in forebrain: sinusoidal respiration), **Hyperventilation**(lesion in midbrain), **Apneusis**(lesion in Pons: inspiratory cramps), **Ataxic breathing** (Lesion in Lower Pons/Upper medulla), **Respiratory arrest**(bilateral lesion in Medulla)
16. **Pupillary Light Responses: Small/reactive**(diffuse forebrain impairment(**metabolic encephalopathy**), pontine injury, sedative drugs(opiates); **Midposition pupils/loss of response**(damage to III at level of midbrain); **Unilateral Pupillary Dilation**(injury to III at exit of brain stem/unilateral compression); **Large/unreactive**(pressure in pretectal area, ex:**pineal tumor**)
17. **Oculomotor responses: Metabolic encephalopathy**(doll's head manoeuvre/Cold/Warm water in ear=>test brainstem; **Right pontine lesion**(no response when try to activate Left vestibular apparatus, Gaze paralysis to the Right); **Midbrain lesion**(III is damaged in Doll's Head manoeuvre, ↓Mesencephalic reticular formation, which organize vertical eye movements)

46. Language and Aphasias

1. Paraphasia – disorderly arrangement of words
2. Neologism – a newly formed, nonexistent words
3. Lexemes- different forms from one word: love,loving, loved...
4. Morpheme- smallest meaningful part of word: dis-like
5. word, grammar, morphology, syntax, phonetics(phonology: **prosody**-pattern of intonation-**Right Hemisphere**)
6. Using language requires complex patterns of info flow thru many parts of the brain.
7. Sounds[7mth]Syllables[8mth]'mama'[1yr]rich phrases[2yrs]correct use/grammar[3yr] – **spontaneous in children**
8. Language use depends on Left hemisphere(even sign lang)- Broca's , Wernicke's
9. Right hemisphere – add emotions to speech. (severe Left lesions- can still sing and learn new songs!)
10. Wernicke's processes auditory info and receives info from **Angular gyrus**,that integrate visual patterns into meaningful info AND outputs to Broca's via **Arcuate Fasciculus.**
11. Reading: input from **Left** visual cortex to Wernicke's
12. Writing: nonverbal meaning→conversion to motor/visual image in Wernicke's→arcuate fasciculus→Broca->**Premotor area** above Broca's
13. Speaking: nonverbal meaning→conversion to acoustic image→arcuate fasciculus→Broca->Motor Cortex
14. Listening: auditory signal→primary auditory cortex →Wernicke's area→evocation of word's meaning in brain near Wernicke's area.
15. Aphasia- disorder of speech,writing(agrahia), reading(alexia): Fluent/ Nonfluent
16. **fluent**: **Wernicke's aphasia**(poor comprehension/fluent word salad); **Transcortical sensory aphasia**(lesion of secondary associated cortex in perisylvian area=>inability to speak spontaneously/deficit of comprehension with normal repetition/naming); **Gerstmann Syndrome**(lesion of angular=>↓reading(visual pattern), acalculia, agraphia); **Conduction aphasia**(lesion of arcuate fasciculus=>normal comprehension but can't repeat)
17. **nonfluent**: **Broca's Aphasia**(or lesion peri-Broca areas: 6,8,9,0,46; comprehension ok/problem with speaking, speak slowly/simply);**Transcortical Motor Aphasia**(damage to left dorsolateral frontal area, Ant & Superior to Broca(word selection); less severe than Broca's aphasia, repetition ok,); **Global Aphasia** (combination of Broca's, Wernicke's, and conduction aphasias)
18. **To test aphasia: speak, repeat, understand** spoken lang, **name** common objects presented visually/tactilely, **Read, Name** written words, **Write.**
19. **Alexia:** disruption in transfer of visual information to the areas of left hemisphere; word blindness(inability to read left visual field); damage in **splenium**(posterior part)
20. **Dyslexia: developmental**(due to abnormal cerebral lateralization(more in left handed)=>improper word-identification, inability to process fast, high-contrast visual stimuli(small cells in LGN of magnocellular layers) and **acquired** (damage to left hemisphere, print-to-sound problems)

47. Mental Illness

1. Impairment of Higher Cerebral Functions:
2. ➔Thought/Volition=>**Schizophrenia**: 10%suicide
3. symptoms: impaired cognition/emotion (↓thought/perception/language/sense of self), hallucinations/delusions, disorganized speech/behaviour/thinking, poor memory/concentration, hygiene neglect.
4. differential diagnosis: encephalitis/meningitis, intoxication(amphetamine/PCP/diphenhydramine), brain tumor, manic(depressive illness)
5. pathogenesis: polygenetic + psychodynamic aspects (?)
6. abnormalities: reduced blood flow to Left Globus Pallidus, No increase in blood flow in frontal lobes during memory test, cortex of medial temporal lobe is thinner and smaller anterior portion of hippocampus, enlarged Lateral/3rd ventricles, Wider Sulci, reduced volume of temporal/frontal lobe.
7. treatment: 2 types of drugs: **Typical** antipsychotics (HALDOL: high affinity to D2-Rs, but SE: blockage of D1/D2-Rs in Basal Ganglia=>Short term hand tremor/muscle rigidity, long term **Tardive Dyskinesia**) and **Atypical** antipsychotics (CLOZAPINE, OLANZAPINE: high affinity for D3/D4 receptors, No side effects in **extrapyramidal system**)
8. **Typical** Antipsychotic Drugs: L-DOPA(↑Dopamine production), AMPHETAMINE(↑release of D), HALOPERIDOL/PERPHENAZINE(block D-receptors), COCAINE/AMPHETAMINE/BENZTROPINE(inhibit reuptake of D to nerve terminals)
9. ➔Mood/Affect=> **Depression/Mania:** onset at 28 in women>men
10. pathogenesis: polygenic+ additional stress(social/health/financial)
11. types: **Major depression**(dysfunction in ability to work/focus/sleep/eat/enjoy), **Dysthymia**(less severe, not disabling long-term chronic symptoms)
12. symptoms: persistent sadness, pessimism, guilt, loss of interest in hobbies, ↓energy, ↓memory, diet abnormalities, *persistent physical symptoms that do not respond to treatment, such as headaches, digestive disorders, chronic pain.*
13. treatment: psychotherapy with antidepressants(MAO inhibitors, Tricyclic antidepressants, Selective serotonin reuptake inhibitor, Electroconvulsive Therapy[causes an epileptic seizure])
14. Prophylactic treatment: Lithium, Carbamazepine, Lamotrigine, Valproate. – **Mood Stabilizers**
15. **Bipolar Disorder:** 'manic-depressive' illness. Cyclic mood changes from high(mania) to low(depression).
16. **Mania:** symptoms: excessive elation, unusual irritability, ↓need for sleep, grandiose notions, ↑talking, ↑sexual desire, poor judgement/increased energy. **Treatment**: typical antipsychotics
17. **Imaging showed:** ↓activity of prefrontal cortex, below the genu in Corpus Callosum in depressive states (↑ in Mania states): the area is important in mood, cause has connections to Amygdala, Hypothalamus, Nucleus accumbens, and NA/5HT/D-ergic systems of brainstem.
18. ➔Language=>Aphasia, dyslexia, alexia
19. ➔Memory/learning=> Mental retardation/Dementia
20. ➔Social behaviour=>Personality disorders.

48. Addiction

1. during past 3 yrs: ↓control,↑withdrawal, ↑dose, behaviour..
2. **bio-psycho-social disease**
3. Serotonin lacking in in patients with addiction
4. Cloninger personality factors: **Type1 addiction:**↓novelty seeking, ↑harm avoidance/reward dependence; **Type2 addiction:**↑novelty seeking, ↓harm avoidance/reward dependence
5. Addictive substances activate: **Brain Reward Centre: Ventral Tegmental Area**[Dopamine]=> =>**Nucleus accumbens/Striatum/Frontal cortex** (motivation centres)
6. Need brain reward system to generate normal behaviour like food/water intake/reproduction
7. Addicts enjoy **a mood change (?)** and turn towards addictive behaviour in uncomfortable situations
8. Short-term positive consequences are remembered better than long-term negative=>repetitive behaviour
9. Society – Addictive, p56-7
10. Drug effects: Sedative, Hallucinogenic, Stimulative=> withdrawal from Stimulative drugs results in sedation,↓BP,bradycardia (no need med help); Withdrawal from Sedative drugs results in excitation, ↑BP, tachycardia, epileptic seizures, psychosis (need med help)
11. **Alcohol detoxification-** 3-8hrs after no alcohol=>Withdrawal(lasts5-7days): nausea trembling, sweating, craving, **delirium,** seizures. Delirium can be fatal. Use BENZODIAZEPINES for detoxification +VitB1(thiamine for Wernicke-Korsakoff syndrome).
12. DIAZEPAM(antiadrenergic,anti-convulsive,anti-psychotic), HALOPERIDOL(anti-psychotic), CLONIDINE(anti-adrenergic)
13. **Opiate detoxification-** COLD: ~GI influenza, meds for symptoms(nausea/diarrhea/Tachycardia,↑BP), 2/3rd days are the worst, Hyposomnia for weeks.; WARM: sub with METHADONE, reducing dose over 3wks, meds for symptoms. Needs long supervision, easy to break off.

49. EEG & Epilepsy

1. Epilepsy – recurrent seizures(hypersynchronous electrical activity)
2. Electroencephalogram- electrodes on scalp to record **beta**(12+hz,Low Amplitude,Over Frontal region in Wake), **alpha**(8-12hz, Over occipital region, in wake/eyes closed), **theta**(4-8Hz, drowsy adults/children, just before sleep), **delta**(4-hz, deep sleep/ encephalopathy).
3. EEG is different at different age: Infant(↑delta), Child(↑theta/delta), Adult(↑alpha/beta, Old(alpha/δ/the)
4. EEG should be symmetrical, if not=>lesions, the slower the waves the bigger the lesion.
5. Sharp waves, spikes-and-wave complexes – Epilepsy
6. Use EEG in : Seizure disorders(to locate lesion), Transient spells, Intracranial disease process, Diffuse disturbances of cerebral function(encephalitis, Creutzfeldt-Jakob disease), Coma, Death.
7. **Epilepsy:** most common neurological disease, happen when seizure threshold is low. **Primary: idiopathic**(genetically low threshold/seizure focus is in deep cerebral structures): **Grand Mal Seizures**(tonic-clonic seizure, tongue biting); **Secondary:** known reason-known focus/region, predict with **aura**(preceding symptoms):**Intracranial**(tumor, vascular, infection)/**Extracranial**(metabolic, anoxia, ↓Glu, drugs).
8. **Positive epileptic symptoms:** sensory(flashes, fear, hear things), Motor(jerking of limb/face)
9. **Negative epileptic symptoms:** sensory(↓brain function), Motor(**Todd Paralysis**)
10. **Tests:** blood, EEG, CAT,MRI,PET. BUT do NOT confirm/rule out Epilepsy
11. Treat with: Anti-epileptic drugs(PHENYTOIN/CARBAMAZEPINE(Na-channel blockers=>↓excitation), BENZODIAZEPINE/BARBITURATES/GABA-ergic(enhance inhibition)) or Neurosurgery
12. Can control seizures by avoiding triggers.
13. **Epileptic status:** when seizures are not self-limiting, and can have one after the other, need ICU

50. Sleep

1. **REM**(paradoxical sleep~wake EEG)-**NREM**(4 stages) cycles, with REM increasing every time
2. regulated by internal clock in SCN, which influences pineal gland(↑melatonin at night).
3. Thalamus/Cortex kept active in wake by **Ascending reticular arousal system**(brainstem,hypothalamus, basal forebrain) with 3 systems of neurons: ACh,5HT,NE.
4. Sleep-promoting agents: Immune-related: IL-1in CSF; Delta sleep-inducing peptide(animals), **Melatonin**(2am max, in nocturnal animals-stimulates wakefulness!); Muramyl peptide from bacterial cell walls, **Adenosine**(rises with wake, declines in sleep).
5. EEG: **synchronized**(neurons around electrode fire at the same time: see in sleep(except REM) when there is no input from Thalamus); **desynchronized**(neuron are not under simultaneous stimulation, Wake)
6. 5 stages of sleep(observe with EEG, $EO_{cular}G$,EMG): NREM1(theta waves), NREM2(spindles+K complex), NREM3(Delta low voltage), NREM4(delta high voltage), REM(beta)
7. Eye movement/respiration/penile erection/HR decreases with NREM stages, ↑↑inREM.
8. However Muscle tone is lowest in REM (paralysis, LMN inhibited)
9. Sensation is vivid but **internally** generated in REM (as opposed to Wake-externally)
10. Dreams – cortical activity in REM: visual/auditory sensations.
11. PET showed in REM **extrastriate cortex**(visual cortex not involved) and **limbic** system is active
12. Both REM and NREM decline with age. NREM peaks at puberty and then falls
13. **Sleep function? Rest theory**(sleep provides fall in neuronal/metabolic activity in NREM), **Behavioural advantage**(out of trouble in sleep), **Maintenance**(rest neurons in NREM, activate some in REM), **Memory processing**(short term consolidated to Long term), **Maturation**(of NS in REM)
14. **Sleep Deprivation:** lethal, execution, tortures=>damages cognitive/mental ability
15. **Cognitive deficit** persists for several days after period of sleep deprivation.
16. **REM** deprivation-↑rebound inREM requirement, but no ↓in cognitive ability as in NREM deprivation
17. Slow waves in NREM originates from rhythmic firing of cortical neurons without input from Thalamic **Relay** nucleus and ARAS, which see as sleep spindles(random thalamic firing in NREM2)/K complexes – associated with ↓sensory input to Thalamus/Cortex
18. At REM onset Cholinergic neurons from brainstem activate LGN of thalamus and Association Visual cortex (occipital cortex), which can be seen as PGO(pontine-geniculate-occipital) waves on EEG. Pontine cholinergic neurons also have synapses on CNIII=>eye movements.
19. Also at REM there is activation of descending Inhibitory Glycinergic nuclei (reticulospinal) that synapse on cranial and motor neurons=>muscle paralysis in REM
20. As REM onsets, firing from **Locus Coeruleus** and **Raphe nuclei** Decreases.
21. Sleep disorders: Insomnia (transient/chronic/drug-induced), **Narcolepsy**(frequent sleep attacks, REM within 10mins, **cataplexy**(sleep-associated paralysis), **hypnagogic hallucinations**(pre-sleep dreams));
22. **Sleep apnea** deprives of sleep and causes daytime sleepiness.
23. **Fatal Familial Insomnia**- atrophy of some thalamic nuclei, ANS malfunction, motor/memory affected – **PRION disease** (infectious proteins)
24. **sleep Apnea:** Obstructive, Central, Mixed=> no NREM3/4, little REM=>sleep deprived, Fast latency.

25. **Parasomnias: Sleepwalking** – usually in NREM4 within 1-2hours of sleep; **Nightmares**(wake up from REM dream), **Sleep Terror**(disturbed sleep while in NREM4=>anxiety,tachycardia,sweating), **Sleep Paralysis**(before of after sleep, normal awareness)
26. sleep disorders with abnormal movements: **Restless leg syndrome**(when sitting/lying down=>delays sleep onset, insomnia), **PeriodicRLS**(during sleep only). **Dream enactment**(in REM incomplete motor inhibition)
27. Motor disorders(tremor/chorea/dystonia/hemiballismus) are inhibited in sleep.

51. Memory Systems

1. **Declarative**(facts in Hippocampal formation/Diencephalon, available to Consciousness) memory.
2. **NonDeclarative** (skills in Supplementary/Premotor cortex/Striatum/Cerebellum/Amygdala, not available to Consciousness) memory.
3. **Intermediate**(seconds)→**Short term**('working memory', minutes), **Long term**(yrs).
4. **Amnesia:** Retrograde(forget all before trauma), Anterograde(can't form new memories after trauma), Transient global(transient cerebral ischemia)
5. **Engram** – envisioned memory trace: Circuit of neurons involved in memory storage undergo **Hebbian** modification to strengthen connections after stimulation.
6. Engrams in brain distributed in neocortex, comprise **association areas** that receive sensory from Visual/auditory/somatosensory cortices and Send it for processing to **medial temporal lobe** in the **hippocampal formation**, which relays back to association areas for memory **consolidation.**
7. Synapses within the Engram show **Synaptic plasticity**
8. **Prefrontal neocortical areas** – Working memory, tags memories with time and place.
9. Case: damage to right thalamus/medial temporal lobe=>anterograde amnesia
10. case: ischemic attack=> bilateral lesions to hippocampus(↓CA1 neuron)=>anterograde amnesia
11. **Hippocampal formation**= dentate gyrus+hippocampus+subiculum
12. **Info flow:** Cortical association area⇔Parahippocampal/Rhinal cortical areas→Dentate gyrus[Mossy fibers]→CA3 Hippocampal cells[Schaffer collateral]→CA1 Hippocampal cells→Subiculum→ **loop** back to Parahippocampal/Rhinal cortical areas to induce **Synaptic plasticity** on structures in the loop.
13. Increased firing(100/s) of CA3 on CA1 neurons increases synaptic efficiency (**long term potentiation** of Glutamatergic synapses on dendritic spines of CA1**).**
14. **LTP** is caused by changes of postsynaptic membrane in CA1: 1st AMPA conductance is increase, 2nd **more AMPA** receptors inserted(↑sensitivity), later **more dendritic spines** formed(↑#of synapses).
15. Mechanism: single impulse only activates AMPA-Na channel, but NMDA is still blocked by Mg^{2+}, a **train** of impulses unblocks NMDA=>Ca influx=> ↑**Protein Kinase C / Ca-Calmodulin dependent protein kinase II** (CAMKII)=>phosphorylation of key membrane proteins, including AMPA.
16. Low frequency firing(1/sec) of CA3 on CA1 causes **Long Term depression** of synaptic activity, which also(like LTP) depends on NMDA activation, BUT low levels of Ca enter the cell=>**phosphatases** active=>dephosphorylation of AMPAR=>internalization=>LTD.
17. LTP/LTD observed in Hippocampus, and Neocortex as well.
18. **Procedural memory of learnt movements: Cerebellum** also show **Synaptic plasticity:** Purkinje cells receive input from **Parallel fiber**(Glutamate on AMPA and metabotropic) in molecular layer and **Climbing fiber**(many excitatory synapses that open Na and Ca channels) from below=> cause LTD in purkinje synapses via reduction of AMPAR by phosphorylation with PKC activated by metabotropic GlutR.
19. **Korsakoff Syndrome:** ↓thiamine in alcoholics=>bilateral loss of cells in dorsomedial thalamus/mammillary bodies.=> confusion. Memory impairment: anterograde/retrograde amnesia.
20. **Electroconvulsive therapy:** for clinical depression, pass current to evoke seizures. May cause amnesia
21. *Dinoflagellate Pfiesteria piscida:* neurotoxin to sea=>skin/inhale=>confusion/↓concentration/ disorientation/memory loss.

52. Aging & Alzheimer's disease

1. dementia- loss of intellectual ability
2. Life expectancy –rising in developed countries, low in Africa due to HIV/AIDS; determined by Socio-economic position. Increase in lifespan also mean ↑% of **senile dementia** and other age-related diseases, like Osteoporosis.
3. age-related Sensory impairments: visual, olfactory, hearing, vestibular, proprioception.
4. age-related Motor impairments: muscle, gait, basal ganglia(Parkinson/Huntington), cerebellum
5. age-related Cognitive impairments: Dementia(**Alzheimer's, Pick's** disease), Personality disturbances.
6. CV disease/stroke ↑ with age.
7. Aging of NS: after 30 brain weight declines, ↓Neuronal size/dendritic arborization/number of synapses, Gyri narrower, sulci/fissure/ventricles/cisterns enlarge=> ↓function
8. **Alzheimer's**: unknown cause of dementia; **Type1**(late onset, 65+), **Type2**(early onset)
9. **3 signs: Neuritic Senile plaques**(extracellular deposits with neuritic/glial processes within central core of **amyloid beta** protein), **Neurofibrillary tangles**(intracellular paired helical filaments), **Granulovacuolar degeneration**(intracellular circular clear zones of cytoplasm(vacuoles)) =>interrupt cell signalling in **CA1**,neocortex, amygdala, basal forebrain, locus coeruleus, raphe nuclei, Olfactory cortex, **basal nucleus of Meynert**, limbic area selectively of NE/Dopamine/ACh-ergic neurons
10. **Amyloid** precursor protein is usually within neuronal cell membrane, cleaved in **Abeta** sequence by **α-secretase** and part released to extracellular fluid, which forms the core of Neuritic Senile Plaques when abnormally cleaved in AD patients by **beta-secretase/γ-secretase** into Abeta1-40/43 segments.
11. Abnormal Abeta segments aggregate into deposits with axon terminals/microglia/astrocytes and cause production of neurofibrillary tangles with help of hyperphosphorylated **Tau proteins**, which normally act in microtubule assembly for axonal transport.
12. 6 stages of Alzheimer's over 20 yrs. p60-12
13. Parkinson's: 60-80yrs, ↓neurons in substantia nigra: loss of pigmentation of substantia nigra, presence of **Lewy** bodies(↑**α synuclein**) within SNc, locus ceruleus, basal nucleus of Meynert, raphe nuclei, cerebral cortex.
14. Huntington's: 50yrs, atrophy of frontal cortices, caudate nuclei, putamen, with ↓GABA and glutamate decarboxylase, **astrogliosis.**
15. Amyotrophic Lateral Sclerosis: 50yrs, gliosis/atrophy of anterior horn cells=> loss of hand motor than legs. Intellect is normal.
16. **Friedreich's Ataxia**: spinocerebellar degeneration, 10-20yrs, atrophy of Dorsal columns, corticospinal tracts, spinocerebellar tracts=>progressive limb ataxia, ↓deep tendon reflex, but Intellect is normal.
17. **Pick's disease:** 40-50yrs, initially ~Alzheimer's: dementia, death in 10yrs, females>males; frontally/temporally localized unilateral Cortical atrophy, surviving neurons accumulate cytoplasmic inclusions (Pick's bodies) composed of **neurofilaments**, ACh-ergic neurons depleted in nucleus of Meynert.
18. **Creutzfeldt-Jakob disease(PRION):** 40-50yrs, incubation of infectious prion 10-30yrs, death within 2yrs of onset, which can be from infection, sporadic, or familial.=>dementia/motor weakness: neuronal loss, astrogliosis, cytoplasmic vacuoles in neurons of cortex/BG(spongiform appearance), amyloid plaques with PrP.
19. **Chromosome 21** – amyloid protein=> Alzheimer's αDown syndrome(trisomy 21)

20. **Progeria:** rapid aging in children. Defective protein that holds nucleus and cell together.

53. Vascular Brainstem Syndromes

1. Brainstem contents: CN nuclei, Red Nucleus, Olive, Raphe n.., Tracts, Reticular formation
2. Diseases of Cranial nerves: **MLF syndrome:** InterNuclear Ophthalmoplegia, lost communication between VI and III, nystagmus in contralateral eye at extreme abduction; Bilateral INO, cannot abduct both eyes, ok convergence. INO/BINO caused by Multiple Sclerosis, Brainstem Infarction/Tumour.
3. Diseases of Cranial nerves: **PPRF Lesion:** ipsilateral conjugate horizontal gaze palsy.
4. Diseases of Cranial nerves: **One and a Half syndrome:** lesion in Pons, unilateral damage to MLF and PPRF, usually from Ischemic/Hemorrhagic stroke of Brainstem, or by Multiple sclerosis(demyelination)
5. Diseases of Cranial nerves: **Facial Palsy**: i)UMN lesion: unilateral Cortical=>contralateral lower facial palsy; ii)LMN lesion (VII)=> ipsilateral full face palsy.
6. Brainstem Syndromes: **Weber's Syndrome:** lesion to posterior midbrain/cerebral peduncle due to infarction of supplying artery (Short penetrating Paramedian branches of Basilar a, or Posterior Cerebral a.)=>↓Substantia nigra(contralateral Parkinsonism), ↓Corticospinal tract(contralateral spastic hemiplegia), ↓Corticobulbar fibers(contralateral facial/hypoglossal paralysis), ↓Oculomotor(ipsilateral+PNS to pupils)
7. Brainstem Syndromes: **Mid-Pontine Syndrome:** lesion to posterior pons due to infarction of 1+ short circumferential branches on one side of the basilar artery=> ↓Corticospinal tract(contralateral spastic hemiplegia), ↓Trigeminal nerve(Ipsilateral hemianesthesia/flaccid paralysis of chewing muscles), ↓Middle Cerebral peduncle(ipsilateral Hemiataxia)
8. Brain Stem Syndromes: **Wallenberg's Syndrome:** stroke in brainstem of Vertebral or PICA=> ↓ALS(contralateral analgesia/thermanesthesia), ↓Central Sympathetic pathway (Ipsilateral Horner's), ↓Nucleus of V(ipsilateral analgesia, thermoanesthesia of face, no corneal reflex), ↓Inferior Cerebellar peduncle(ipsilateral ataxia).

BONUS: Relevant topics in Anatomy

53. ANS General Overview

1. Parasympathetic system –NO innervation to body **wall**.
2. Referred pain – Somatic and Visceral **a**fferents enter the spinal cord at the same level and a **dorsal root ganglion**. Brain cannot distinguish between the two and always makes us feel the somatic pain. The only difference, when pain is caused by visceral afferents (travel with **sympathetic fibers**), we feel it as dull and diffused, when, on the other hand, pain is from somatic afferents, we feel it as sharp and localized. Referred pain is caused by anoxia/ischemia, distension, inflammation, or spasmodic contraction of muscles of **visceral organs**.
3. SNS ganglia are in the Sympathetic Chain Ganglia that run parallel to the spinal cord.
    Cervical and Sacral ganglia only have Grey rami communicantes and NO white RC!
4. ALL **sympathetic** preganglionic fibers originate in the **lateral horn** at the level of T1-L2 vertebra.
5. PNS ganglia are located close to the target organs, such as heart, intestine.
6. ALL **parasympathetic** preganglionic fibers originate from brain stem (3,5,7,9,10) and **lateral** horn at the level of S2-S4 sacral vertebrae.

54. ANS of Head Neck.

1. "Head" contains **only 6 ganglia** (extraaxial): 2 sensory(V,VII) + 4 Parasympathetic(Ciliary, PT, Submandibular, Otic).
2. **SNS** for head and neck exit from T1/T2 ascend to Cervical ganglion, from where postganglionic fibers follow carotid arteries (**carotid plexus**) with some following cranial nerves (ex. Deep Petrosal nerve)
3. Parasympathetics exit with CNIII, VII, IX, X and from S2-S4.
    a. **Pupil constriction:** Edinger-Westphal→III→branch to Inferior Oblique→Ciliary Ganglion→**Short Ciliary** nerves→Pupil Constrictors +Ciliary body.
    b. **Tears/mucus:** Superior Salivatory n of Pons→VII→Greater Petrosal nerve→nerve of pterygoid canal→Pterygopalatine ganglion →Greater/Lesser palatine nerves→Nasopalatine nerve(**V2**) [**communicating nerve**]Lacrimal n.(**V1**)
    c. **Saliva:** Superior salivatory n in Pons→VII→Chorda Tympani→Lingual nerve(V3)→Submandibular ganglion→Lingual nerve→Submandibular/Sublingual glands
    d. **Saliva:** Inferior salivatory n in medulla→IX→Lesser petrosal nerve→Otic ganglion→Auriculotemporal nerve→Parotid gland
    e. **GI glands/motility/lung/heart:** Dorsal motor nucleus in medulla→X
4. **NOTE:** the only time PNS and SNS run together is when Deep Petrosal nerve and Greater Petrosal nerve run together in the **Pterygoid canal.**
5. NOTE: Chorda tympani runs across tympanic membrane/crosses malleolus.
6. NOTE: Chorda tympani cares special motor(PNS to submandibular ganglion) and special sensory (taste from anterior 2/3 of tongue)

NEUROSCIENCE: The Most Rapid Review Of All Topics

55. Overview of Cranial Nerves

1. **Olfactory/Optic/***Oculomotor***/Trochlear/Trigeminal/Abducens/*** Facial***/Vestibulocochlear/ *** Glossopharyngeal***/*** Vagus***/Accessory spinal/Hypoglossal**.
2. Cranial Vault= Anterior[Lesser wing of Sphenoid]Middle$_{II-VI}$[Petrous ridge]Posterior
3. Openings in cranium: Optic canal, Superior Orbital Fissure(III, IV,V1,VI), Foramen Rotundum(V2), Foramen Ovale(V3), Internal Acustic Meatus(VII,VIII), Jugular Foramen (IX,X,XI), Hypoglossal canal(XII).
4. **Parasympathetic** ganglia(4): Ciliary(III→V1), Pterygopalatine(VII→V2/V1), Submandibular(VII→V3), Otic(IX→V3).
5. NOTE: VII passes through Parotid gland, but does NOT innervate it.
6. The latter three supply 'lubricating' **glands**: Lacrimal, Submandibular/Sublingual, Parotid.
7. **V**: ophthalmic$_1$ + maxillary$_2$ + mandibular$_3$ **meet in Trigeminal Ganglion**
8. **Sympathetic** system supplies 'sweat' glands.
9. **VII**: sensory from Ant2/3 tongue, outer ear/eardrum.

Ptosis: 2 reasons: ↓Sympathetics(partial ptosis, **Horner** syndrome) or ↓III

56. Cranial Nerves V and VII

1. **V: Somatic** motor: "Mast MATT", **Parasympathetic** postganglionic motor from Ciliary$_{Edinger-Westphal}$/Pterygopalatine$_{Superior\ Salivatory}$/Submandibular$_{Superior\ Salivatory}$/Otic$_{Inferior\ Salivatory}$ **ganglia**.
2. **V: Sensory**: from Face, 2/3SCALP, 2/3Tongue(NOT taste!), External Acoustic meatus, Nasal/Oral cavities, **Paranasal** cavities.
3. **Pupil constriction**: Edinger-Westphal→III→branch to Inferior Oblique→Ciliary Ganglion→**Short Ciliary** nerves→Pupil Constrictors +Ciliary body.
4. **Tears/mucus**: Superior Salivatory n of Pons→VII→petrosal nerve→nerve of pterygoid canal→Pterygopalatine ganglion→Greater/Lesser palatine nerves, Nasopalatine nerve, Lacrimal n.
5. **Saliva**: Superior salivatory n in Pons→VII→Chorda Tympani→Lingual nerve(V3)→Submandibular ganglion→Lingual nerve→Submandibular/Sublingual glands
6. **Saliva**: Inferior salivatory n in medulla→IX→tympanic/lesser petrosal branches→Otic ganglion→Auriculotemporal nerve→Parotid gland
7. **V1 splits into**: NFL: Nasociliary(**Long Ciliary**-Sympathetics), Frontal(→supraorbital/supratrochlear), Lacrimal
8. **V2 splits into**: Zygomatic + Infraorbital(P/Med/Ant Superior Alveolar)
9. **V3 splits into**: Motor, Auriculotemporal+Inferior alveolar+Lingual
10. **VII: Somatic** motor(Stylomastoid foramen-through Parotid gland): to facial muscles+ Stylohyoid/Posterior Digastric/Stapedius, **Parasympathetic** preganglionic to PT ganglion and Submandibular ganglion.
11. **VII: Sensory**: 2/3Tongue – TASTE, somatic to small area of auricle
12. **VII**: Temporal, Zygomatic **branch**, Buccal **branch**, Mandibular **branch**, Cervical, Posterior Auricular.
13. **Geniculate Ganglion** – sensory somatic ganglion of VII

57. Face & Scalp

1. **Trigeminal: Ophthalmic**(5:Supraorbital, Supratrochlear, Lacrimal, Infratrochlear, External Nasal)
2. **Trigeminal: Maxillary**(3: Zygomaticotemporal, Zygomaticofacial, Infraorbital)
3. **Trigeminal: Mandibular**(3: Auriculotemporal, Buccal, Mental)
4. *Facial Arteries(4): Infratrochlear(IntCarotid), Infraorbital(Maxillary), Transverse facial(Superficial Temporal), Facial(ExtCarotid).
5. **Danger area of the face:** around the nose: Ophthalmic veins+Pterygoid Venous Plexus=>**Cavernous Sinus**(encloses III, IV, V1/2, VI) – affected by infection.
6. Facial Muscles(**VII,** Bell's palsy): Frontalis, Orbicularis oculi, Levator labii superioris alaeque nasi, Levator labii superioris, Zygomaticus minor/major ☺, Buccinator, Risorius⑩, Orbicularis oris, Depressor anguli oris☹, Depressor labii inferioris, Mentalis, Platisma, Auricularis, Occipitalis.
7. Parotid duct penetrates Buccinator and opens at 2nd molar maxillary tooth.
8. **Facial CNVII:** 5: Temporal+Zygomatic+Buccal+Mandibular+Cervical branches
9. **SCALP:** skin-Connective tissue(dense)-Aponeurosis-**Loose Connective tissue-**Periosteum
10. Infection in Loose connective tissue can move to Dural Sinuses via **Emissary veins→Diploic veins→Emissary veins→dural sinus**
11. *SCALP Arteries(5): Supraorbital/Supratrochlear(IntCarotid), Superficial temporal/Occipital/ Posterior Auricular(Ext Carotid)

58. Nasal cavity, Pterygopalatine fossa

1. bones: vomer, Inferior concha, Maxilla, Ethmoid, Lacrimal
2. Lacrimal Duct drains to Inferior Meatus
3. Semilunar hiatus – in Middle meatus, drains Frontal sinus, Maxillary sinus
4. Bulla Ethmoidalis – contain/drains middle ethmoidal sinus
5. Posterior Ethmoidal sinus (close to **CNII**) drains to Superior meatus; Anterior Ethmoidal sinus to middle meatus
6. Nasal arteries anastomose in **Locus Kiesselbach** (Little's area)
7. arteries for nasal cavity – from Maxillary: Palate$_{Palatine}$/Teeth$_{alveolar}$
8. Pterygopalatine fossa: accommodates PT ganglion→lacrimal gland/all other glands in the area
9. PT fossa openings: Foramen Rotundum/Pterygoid Canal/Pharyngeal Canal^{Post}, Infraorbital fissure^{Ant}, Greater/Lesser palatine foramena^{Inf}, Pterygomaxillary fissure^{Lat}, Sphenopalatine foramen^{Med}.
10. Gag Reflex: IX-brainstem-X
11. Cough: IX in larynx/trachea-brainstem-X

59. Infratemporal Fossa

2. Ramus of mandible-Styloid process-Lateral Pterygoid plate-Maxilla
3. Contents: Parotid gland, V3, Maxillary artery, Pterygoid plexus of veins, Muscles of mastication.
4. Temporal bone: Mastoid+Styloid+Squamous+Tympanic+Petrous+Zygomatic
5. Sphenoid bone: Greater wing+Lesser Wing+Pterygoid process
6. Muscles of Mastication(**V3**): **Closing**(Temporalis(retracts), Masseter, **Medial** Pterygoid(sidewise)), **Opening(Lateral** Pterygoid(2 heads; protrude)
7. **Mandibular (V3):** MOTOR: **Mast MATT**: muscles of Mastication(**4**), Mylohyoid(from **posterior** trunk), Ant Belly Digastric, Tensor tympani, Tensor Veli Palatini.
8. **Mandibular (V3):** SENSORY(**4**): Auriculotemporal+Lingual(Chorda tympani!)+Inferior Alveolar+ Buccal(from **anterior** trunk).
9. **TMJ**(temporomandibular): Capsule+ Lateral TM lig+**Spheno**mandibular Lig+**Stylo**mandibular lig
10. TMJ: Anterior Tubercle from Zygomatic process prevents dislocation
11. **Middle Meningeal** artery from the Maxillary artery (α epidural hematoma @pterion)
12. **Maxillary** artery: **4** branches to foramena: Middle meningeal, Anterior Tympanic, Accessory Meningeal, Inferior Alveolar.
13. **Maxillary** artery: **4** branches to muscles: Masseteric, Deep Temporal, Pterygoid, Buccal
14. **Maxillary** artery=>Pterygopalatine fossa(through pterygomaxillary fissure): **4** branches: Descending Palatine, Posterior Superior Alveolar, Infraorbital, Sphenopalatine.

60. Orbit and Eye

1. Bones forming the orbit: Frontal+Zygomatic+Maxillary, and Sphenoid/Ethmoid/Palatine/Lacrimal
2. NOTE: 3 foramena on the face for each branch of V: Supra-orbital foramen(V1), Infraorbital foramen(V2), Mental foramen(V3).
3. Orbicularis Oculi: Palpebral+Orbital+Lacrimal$_{tear\ drainage}$
4. Orbicularis Oculi opposed by **Levator palpebrae superioris(III), Tarsalis**(SNS, smooth muscle)
5. 4 Sinuses(empty space/mucosal membrane): Maxillary, Frontal, Ethmoid, Sphenoid$_{next\ to\ pituitary\ gland}$
6. Nasal Cavity: 3 Meatuses: Superior/Middle/Inferior, divided by 2 Conchas: Middle/Inferior (+Superior)
7. Tears drain via Lacrimal sac→Nasolacrimal duct→INFERIOR Meatus.
8. Eye muscles: Inferior Oblique/Inferior rectus/Medial rectus/Superior rectus (III), Superior Oblique(IV), Lateral Rectus (VI)
9. All eye muscle (Except Inferior Rectus) originate from Common tendinous ring.
10. **H-test**: goal is to isolate and test for specific eye muscles: medial gaze for obliques; lateral gaze for Sup/Inf rectuses
11. If III is down: ptosis + lateral/downward gaze (IV+VI)
12. If IV is down on down on one side: cannot go down the stairs normally: help with ipsilateral Sternocleidomastoid to use ipsilateral VI instead. Gaze is NORMAL otherwise
13. If VI is down: gaze is medial
14. Arteries of the eye: Internal Carotid→Ophthalmic→**Central a. of Retina**, Supraorbital, Lacrimal, Ciliary +branches to Ethmoidal sinus.
15. Vein of the eye: connect with **Cavernous sinus**(via Superior/Inferior Ophthalmic vein)
16. All branches of V1 are in the orbit: $N_{asocilliary}F_{rontal}L_{acrimal}$
17. NOTE: V2 has Naso<u>palatine</u>
18. Corneal Reflex: Touch Cornea-**V1**-Brainstem-**VII**-Blink(Orbicularis oculi)
19. Accomodation: See object approaching/moving away-**II**-Brainstem-Adjust Lens shape/Amount of light(**PSN with III**, on Ciliary muscles/Pupillary constrictors)
20. Pupillary light reflex: same as above only isolate **Constrictor Pupillae**
21. Startling reflex: See object coming-**II**-brainstem-**VII**-blink

61. Triangles of the neck

2. **Posterior** triangle borders: SternoCleidoMastoid-Middle 3rd Clavicle-Trapezius.
3. Inferior belly of omohyoid divides Posterior triangle into **Occipital & Supraclavicular**
4. Content of posterior triangle: ^{Post}Splenius Capitis, Levator Scapulae, Post/Med/Ant scalene^{Ant} +External Jugular + Sensory cervical plexus.
5. **Cervical plexus SENSORY Nerves** exit from posterior triangle: ^{S}Lesser Occipital, Great Auricular, Transverse Cutaneous, Supraclavicular^I. +XI, +Brachial Plexus(between Ant & Med scalene)
6. NOTE: 2 Sensori dorsal rami: Greater Occipital + Third Occipital.
7. **Anterior** triangle: Digastric$_{mandible+P\ digastric+A\ digastric}$ + Submental$_{hyoid+2A\ Digasrics}$ + Carotid$_{Lateral\ to\ Sup\ Omohyoid}$ + Muscular triangles$_{Medial\ to\ Sup\ Omohyoid}$.
8. **Jugular veins:** External(posterior triangle), Internal(behind SCM), Anterior(Muscular triangle)
9. Deep Cervical Fascia: Investing layer (Pretracheal$_{recur\ laryngeal}$/Prevertebral$_{phrenic}$ +carotid sheath$_{vagus}$).
10. **Cervical Plexus: C1-C4:** MOTOR to Infrahyoid/Prevertebral muscles of neck+Diaphragm.
11. Ansa cervicalis – motor branches
12. **Subclavian Artery**: **Internal Thoracic+Vertebral Artery+Thyrocervical trunk**(^{I}Suprascapular/Superficial Cervical/Inferior Thyroid^S) + ^{2}**Costocervical trunk**(Deep cervical/Superior Intercostal)+ ^{3}**Dorsal Scapular.**
13. **Common carotid:** from subclavian on the Right; Aortic arch on the Left.
14. Common carotid= **Internal Carotid**(!no neck branches!) + **External Carotid**(^{I}Superior Thyroid/Ascending Pharyngeal/Lingual/Occipital/Facial/Posterior Auricular/Maxillary/Superficial Temporal(transverse facial)^S)
15. **Thyroid-** 2 lobes connected by isthmus (2/3 tracheal rings): 2 arteries + 3 veins(Superior+Medial to Internal Jugular Vein, Inferior to Brachiocephalic vein).

62. Autonomics of Abdomen

1. ANS: **cardiac/smooth** muscles and **glands.**
2. *Take a look at Netter's plate **324**
1. **T1-T4** sympathetic: postganglionic fibers to **Superficial** and **Deep PLEXI** on aorta
2. **T5-T9** sympathetics: combine to **Greater Splanchnic Nerve,** which synapse in **Celiac GANGLION**
3. **T10-11** sympathetics: combine to **Lesser Splanchnic Nerve,** which synapse in **Aorticorenal Ganglion** and **Superior Mesenteric ganglion**
4. **T12** sympathetics: combine to **Least Splanchnic Nerve,** which synapse in **Superior Mesenteric ganglion.**
5. **L1-L2** sympathetics: combine to **Lumbar Splanchnics,** part of which synapse in **Inferior Mesenteric Ganglion;** and the other part: **pre**ganglionic fibers form **Superior Hypogastric PLEXUS**, which divides to **left/right hypogastric NERVE**
3. L/R Hypogastric nerves combine with **Sacral Splanchnics**(sympathetics from sacral ganglia) and **S2-S4 Parasympathetics** into **Inferior pelvic plexus**
4. Vagus nerve travels **through** Celiac and Superior Mesenteric ganglia **without synapsing**
5. Vagus nerve innervates foregut/midgut
6. S2-S4 Parasympathetics innervate hindgut

63. Pelvic Vessels & Nerves.

1. External Iliac artery – supplies the lower limb
2. Internal Iliac artery(Ant/Post) – supplies pelvis/perineum
3. Posterior trunk(of IIA): Iliolumbar+Lateral Sacral+**Superior Gluteal**(in V(lumbosacral trunk & S1 of sacral plexus), superiorly to Piriformis)
4. Anterior trunk(of IIA): Umbilical(Superior Vesicular)+Obturator+Inferior Vesicular+Middle Rectal + **Internal Pudendal**(travels around **Spinous ligament)** **+Inferior Gluteal**(inferiorly to Piriformis)
5. Sacral Plexus: Superior Gluteal n(above piriformis->sup/med gluteal muscles), Inferior Gluteal n(below piriformis->inferior gluteal muscle), Nerve to Piriformis, Sciatic, Post Femoral Cutaneous, **Pudendal**(S2,3,4))
6. TURP(transurethral prostate resection) – try to preserve prostate capsule – contains Parasympathetics for erectile tissue.
7. Lymphatic drainage: follow the arteries.
8. Lymphatic drainage of uterus: upper part(fundus) to Lumbar nodes(with ovarian a), Lower part +Upper vagina to Internal Iliac nodes, lower vagina to inguinal nodes.
9. Lymphatic drainage of anal canal: above pectinate line to Internal Iliac nodes; below pectinate line to Superficial inguinal nodes

64. Development: Blastocyst&Bilaminar disk. Gastrulation/Somites

1. Morula=Zona pellucida&Trophoblast + Inner cell mass – 12-16 cells
2. Cavity forms in morula by day 5=>**Blastocyst**
3. Blastocyst= Trophoblast + ICM(**Hypoblast**(endoderm)&**Epiblast**(ectoderm))
4. NOTE: Cells get smaller in size with each duplication (**quantitative duplication**) because of tough Zona pellucida that does not allow cell growth.
5. During implantation: **Epiblast** cells spread forming new cavity – **amniotic**
6. During implantation: **Hypoblast** cells spread replacing blastocystic cavity with **1° yolk sac.**
7. Plane of connection between epiblast and hypoblast is called **bilaminar disk**
8. **Primary mesoderm (extra**embryonic) forms from **endodermal** cells and fills the space **between** cytotrophoblast and 2 cavities so that there is no contact between initial hypoderm/epiblast and trophoblasts
9. Within the formed mesoderm layer **clefts** begin to appear and fuse together forming **chorionic** cavity.
10. Chorionic cavity pushes the mesodermal cells towards trophoblast&amniotic cavity (**somatic mesoderm**) and towards the yolk sac (**splanchnic mesoderm**)
11. Chorion wall is made up of: somatic mesoderm-cytotrophoblasts-syncytiotrophoblast
12. **Buccopharyngeal membrane** –future site of mouth.
13. Chorionic villi – cytotrophoblastic projections into syncytiotrophoblast.
14. Chorionic villi – 1° (only cytotrophoblasts within syncytiotrophoblasts), 2° (somatic mesoderm moves into the villi), 3° (capillaries [with fetal blood] form).
15. Maternal blood – between the villi.
16. **Gastrulation – tri**laminar disk formation. (3rd week)
17. Epiblast thickens at **caudal end** forming **primitive streak.**
18. **Secondary mesoderm (intra**embryonic) forms from **epiblast** cells from the primitive streak between ectoderm and endoderm (COMPARE to point 8!)
19. (NOTE: Epiblast also forms **embryonic** endoderm (according to notes))
20. Cells from rostral portion of primitive streak form notochordal process starting at **primitive pit.**
21. Notochord grows between ectoderm&endoderm until it hit the buccopharyngeal membrane.
22. 3 parts of embryonic mesoderm (with respect to notochord): paraxial mesoderm (somites), intermediate mesoderm, lateral mesoderm (coelomic space)
23. SACROCOCCYGEAL teratoma – remnants of **primitive streak,** tumour with all three germ layers.
24. Notochord induces **neural plate** formation from **ectoderm**
25. Neural plate folds into **neural tube** with **neural crest** remnants (Spina Bifida)
26. Vasculogenesis (individual vessel formation) VS Angiogenesis (networks formation)
27. Blood forms 2 weeks later after vessel formation!
28. There are 2 embryonic arteries + 1 umbilical vein = in umbilical cord.
29. Lateral folding impinges part of the yolk sac-GI lumen.
30. GASTROSCHISIS/ ECTOPIA CORDIS – incomplete fusion of lateral folds.
31. SIRENOMELIA – faulty gastrulation

65. Development of Brain

1. Neural tube – CNS; Neural Crest cells – PNS(sensory ganglia, Pia/Arachnoid)
2. Neural tube closes by 4th week: Spina Bifidas, **Meningoencephalocele**(cranium bifidum), **Anencephaly**
3. Prosencephalon(tele- diencephalon) -Mesencephalon-Rhombencephalon(met-,myelencephalon)
4. Holoprosencephaly – no cleavage of the forebrain, undivided lateral ventricle.
5. Congenital hydrocephalus : communicative/non-communicative
6. Hydranencephaly – obstruction of Internal Carotid artery: massive cranium, no cerebral hemispheres
7. 3 brain flexures: Midbrain (mesencephalic) flexure, Pontine flexure$^{convec\ ventrally}$, Cervical flexure^{dorsal}
8. Pituitary gland: Rathke's pouch from ectoderm →**Adenohypophysis**^{ANT}; Neuroectodermal downgrowth from diencephalons→**Neurohypophysis**^{POST}
9. **Craniopharyngiomas** – benign/functional tumors in remnants of hypophyseal diverticulum(Rathke's)
10. **Pharyngeal hypophysis** – accessory anterior pituitary tissue on the path of Rathke's diverticulum.
11. **Arnold-Chiari Malformation** – cerebellum/medulla through foramen magnum to vertebral canal.

66. Development of Ear

1. **1st Pharyngeal arch** (1st of 6 Branchial$_{pharyngeal}$ arches) mesodermal tissue that gives rise to Mandible and all muscles attached to it (exceptions?) + Malleus/Incus and their muscle, Tensor Tympani
2. NOTE: Stapes develops from 2nd Pharyngeal arch along with Hyoid bone.
3. Ear parts: Helix/Antihelix, Tragus/Antitragus, Concha, Lobule
4. NOTE: Incisura Terminalis – area in Anterior to Tragus – no cartilage, can cut in surgery.
5. Sensory Innervation of Ear: C2/3$_{Great\ Auricular\ nerve}$, V3$_{Auriculotemporal}$, VII, IX, X=> ear can hurt for many reasons(tooth abscess/tongue/TMJ^{V3}, cancer of larynx^X, middle ear infection^{IX}, Damage to Cervical spine$^{C2/3}$: all give **otalgia** (earache)
6. NOTE: When Auriculotemporal nerve branches of V3 it splits around Middle Meningeal Artery.
7. NOTE: Infection can travel up the **Eustachian tube** (pharyngotympanic tube) to middle ear and from there spread to **Mastoid air cells**.
8. **Nervus Intermedius** – Sensory and PNS component of VII
9. Tensor Tympani muscle – pulls on Malleus to tense the tympanic membrane, innervated by **V3**
10. Stapedius – pulls on Stapes, to decrease amplification of sound, innervated by **VII**
11. NOTE: **Chorda tympani** of VII is on the tympanic side; **Tympanic plexus** of IX is on promontory (gives rise to lesser petrosal)
12. **EAR:** External ear is formed from **fusion** of 6 hillocks around the 1st Branchial groove: 3 from 1st arch, 3 from 2nd.
13. **External** acoustic meatus : from extension of 1st pharyngeal groove (recanalized meatal plug)
14. **Tympanic** membrane – from ALL 3 layers: endo/meso/ecto derm
15. **Internal ear** and all its structures form from ectodermal **otic vesicles** (starts as otic placode→otic pit→vesicle)
16. **Middle ear space** is formed from 1st Pharyngeal **POUCH**
17. Meckel's$_{Malleus/Incus}$ cartilage(1st Arch); Reichert's$_{Stapes}$ cartilage(2nd arch)

67. Development of Eye

1. **1st arch Syndromes:** Treacher-Collins, Robin: Underdeveloped lower jaw(**micrognathia**)=>little mouth volume=>tongue pushed upwards=>cleft palate. Also ↓other 1st Pharyngeal arch derivatives: Malleus/Incus=> hearing problems
2. **EYE:** forms as **optic groves** from neural tube become **optic diverticula**(vesicle+stalk) that shapes into **optic cup** and induces ectoderm to form **lens placode.** Further invagination of Optic Cup forms **retinal fissure**(choroid fissure) that encloses **Hyaloid artery**$_{=>central\ artery\ of\ retina}$ and **fuses** around it.
3. If retinal fissure does not **fuse**=>COLOBOMA of the iris (keyhole pupil)
4. Retina develops from outer layer of optic cup (neural layer from inner)=> two layers fuse=>easy for detachment.
5. Optic nerve develops from Optic stalk
6. Distal Hyaloid artery degenerates after 6 weeks=> lens becomes avascular.
7. **Choroid/Sclera** – from Mesoderm
8. **Cornea** – from 2 layers: ectoderm$_{epithelium}$/mesoderm$_{fibrous}$/neural crest cells$_{endothelium}$
9. Congenital anIRIdia – no iris, arrest of optic cup development.
10. Congenital aPHAKia – no lens, failure of lens placode formation
11. Congenital Cataract – maternal rubella=> lens opaque at birth
12. Persistent Hyaloid artery – interfere with vision
13. Microphthalmia – small eye, maybe due to Rubella
14. Anophthalmia – no eye
15. Cryptophthalmos – no palpebral fissure (eyelids did not separate at 26wk)

NEUROSCIENCE: The Most Rapid Review Of All Topics